Yoga-Pilates

Yoga-Pilates

A unique blend of two classic disciplines, showing more than 70 poses in over 300 easy-to-follow step-by-step photographs

JONATHAN MONKS

southwater

This edition is published by Southwater, an imprint of Anness Publishing Ltd, Hermes House, 88–89 Blackfriars Road, London SE1 8HA; tel. 020 7401 2077; fax 020 7633 9499

www.southwaterbooks.com; www.annesspublishing.com

If you like the images in this book and would like to investigate using them for publishing, promotions or advertising, please visit our website www.practicalpictures.com for more information.

UK agent: The Manning Partnership Ltd; tel. 01225 478444; fax 01225 478440; sales@manning-partnership.co.uk
UK distributor: Book Trade Services; tel. 0116 2759086; fax 0116 2759090; uksales@booktradeservices.com;
    exportsales@booktradeservices.com
North American agent/distributor: National Book Network; tel. 301 459 3366; fax 301 429 5746; www.nbnbooks.com
Australian agent/distributor: Pan Macmillan Australia; tel. 1300 135 113; fax 1300 135 103; customer.service@macmillan.com.au
New Zealand agent/distributor: David Bateman Ltd; tel. (09) 415 7664; fax (09) 415 8892

Publisher: Joanna Lorenz
Managing Editor: Judith Simons
Project Editor: Katy Bevan
Photography: John Freeman,
    assisted by Alex Dow

Make-up: Bettina Graham
Models: Carly Milnes and Lesley Portner
Designer: Adelle Morris
Editorial Reader: Alison Bolus
Production Controller: Darren Price

ETHICAL TRADING POLICY
At Anness Publishing we believe that business should be conducted in an ethical and ecologically sustainable way, with respect for the environment and a proper regard to the replacement of the natural resources we employ.

As a publisher, we use a lot of wood pulp to make high-quality paper for printing, and that wood commonly comes from spruce trees. We are therefore currently growing more than 750,000 trees in three Scottish forest plantations: Berrymoss (130 hectares/320 acres), West Touxhill (125 hectares/305 acres) and Deveron Forest (75 hectares/185 acres). The forests we manage contain more than 3.5 times the number of trees employed each year in making paper for the books we manufacture.

Because of this ongoing ecological investment programme, you, as our customer, can have the pleasure and reassurance of knowing that a tree is being cultivated on your behalf to naturally replace the materials used to make the book you are holding.

Our forestry programme is run in accordance with the UK Woodland Assurance Scheme (UKWAS) and will be certified by the internationally recognized Forest Stewardship Council (FSC). The FSC is a non-government organization dedicated to promoting responsible management of the world's forests. Certification ensures forests are managed in an environmentally sustainable and socially responsible way. For further information about this scheme, go to www.annesspublishing.com/trees

A CIP catalogue record for this book is available from the British Library.

PUBLISHER'S NOTE
The author and publisher have made every effort to ensure that all instructions contained within this book are accurate and safe, and cannot accept liability for any resulting injury, damage or loss to persons or property, however it may arise. If you do have any special needs or problems, consult your doctor or a physiotherapist. This book cannot replace medical consultation and should be used in conjunction with professional advice.

CONTENTS

FOREWORDS

Balance: it's one of the things that we crave for in our lives. A balanced diet, a balanced chequebook – even a set of balanced front tyres on our car. But, what the vast majority of us don't realize is that our body's movements need balance as well. Without this balance the muscles, nerves and joints that produce our movements become overloaded, and, given time, they can begin to break down and lead to pain.

Any of you who have suffered a problem that began slowly and insidiously will know what I mean – and there are a lot of you out there. As a physiotherapist, I identify and treat these movement problems all the time and spend a large proportion of my treatments educating my clients in the right way of moving. However, when Jonathan came along I was unprepared for the level of insight and awareness he had into the workings of his own body, and also the degree of control that he had when performing his unique form of yoga. The teacher became the pupil when I went to one of his classes.

So read this book and feel inspired to learn how to gain more control of your body. I am proud of having had an input towards helping the most balanced man I know.

GREG RYAN MCSP SRP
(Chartered Physiotherapist) Co-Founder of Health and Fitness Solutions Ltd.

Having spent most of my adult life outside my body, unconfident of its latent power and sensuality and unawake to its expressiveness and natural grace, encountering Jonathan Monks was nothing less than a revelation.

He often asks during his extraordinary classes, "Where are you?" The question is both pragmatic and philosophical. As his student I am encouraged to say in response, "Here, in my body."

The experience is one of intense discovery and delight – an emergence into oneself. The teaching is dynamic, uncompromising and provocative, and never less than exhilarating.

The multivarious asanas (postures), seamlessly practised, lead my body into its centre, its own heart. I begin to learn through Jonathan's technique and perception that there is a natural length and breadth to be unveiled by each of us as we live each day. Our shape changes, we become longer, leaner, sexier, we become alive to ourselves.

The process is unique, authentic and forged by Jonathan Monks' own adventuring on the mat. He makes you sweat diamonds and leap beyond your limitations.

And then, as the class lie down in the final stillness and afterglow, we are gently returned to the original question. Where we are is here, unadulterated, open. And smiling.

Jonathan is a remarkable teacher and I am grateful that he is helping me to stretch my body towards the confidence and strength it has lacked for so long.

GREG HICKS
(Actor, Royal Shakespeare Company)

INTRODUCTION

Yoga and Pilates are both usually regarded as separate disciplines, and are practised as such. Normally, time is spent defining their individual theories and their origins to give them a distinct identity. This provides us with security in that we know what we practise; it's something definable and safe. The fact is, however, that each discipline you learn is as individual as the teacher you learn it from. It may be yoga of one of the many different varieties or Pilates from a highly qualified instructor, but it is still about feelings that are particular to each individual, and the responses that they will have to a given set of physical feelings.

This book is all about you, your body and how you relate to it. There is no in-depth history, proof of origins, or philosophy. In this book I offer you a method by which to find sensations in your body along with opportunities to feel and respond to them. It will allow you to create your own personal style – a personal form of exercise that you can take up, adapt and practise, wherever you are, whatever you are doing.

WHY THIS BOOK WORKS

The information in this book can work only if you feel your body and begin to use it properly. This means that you have to practise regularly, taking an interest in what you are doing when you are doing it, not just going through the motions with the aim that all will be fine in the end. Pay attention to how you feel when you practise; are you a morning or evening person? Do you need twenty minutes practice every day or a thorough hour every other day? Only you can truly say what feels best for you.

I offer the contents of this book to young and old alike, but always with the aim of getting you to understand your body from the inside. When this happens I have seen long-term neck pain disappear in five minutes. I have seen better posture emerge through simple feeling and understanding in half an hour, and clients have dropped a clothes size in between three and six months. However, this is somewhat irrelevant for two reasons. The first is that these people have decided to practise because they enjoy it. They have changed their diet and drinking habits because they have felt they wanted to. They have grown into their bodies and now enjoy life through their bodies. The second reason why other people's stories are irrelevant is because they are not you. Be your own story: be your own body. Everything you've been looking for – the body beautiful – literally lies at your fingertips.

HOW TO USE THIS BOOK

Read this book and, when you are ready, try it out and have a go. Try to exercise every day, even if it is only for a short period of time – little and often is best to start with. However, if you don't understand anything, take the time to reread that section, and break down the sentences until you

left It's hard to know where to begin on the journey of discovering your body, so I suggest you start off with what you truly know and feel. Take some time to discover how you use the ground beneath you, for in that knowledge you can unearth how and why you move.

can identify the body parts and movements I describe. You will find no visualizations or imaginative descriptions to aid you, since all this does is push your concentration farther inside your mind, the opposite direction of where all the action is actually going on: inside your body. Go through the first section, Core Strength, and become familiar with those sensations before you move on to the main postures.

Solid Grounding is dedicated to reflecting on the imperfections of your body, and various ways of dealing with them. If you use this information in combination with the rest of the section on Core Strength, you may find the rare combination of stability and balance that solves your particular problems.

The section on sequences provides some ideal warm-up routines for you to begin with, but once again, be honest about the sensations your body is registering. If you find something hard work, try the easier option, and perhaps try it again the following day until it becomes easier. If you find it too easy, then spend more time in each posture, or try the harder option, extending your sequences for as long as you can manage to build stamina. Take a deep breath and begin your journey towards a stronger, leaner body.

A NOTE ON BREATHING

The subject of breathing fills many books. Such an important issue demands great attention. So how should you breathe? You have done a great job until now, because you are still here, but can you answer the questions, "How do I breathe?" and, "Where do I breathe from and to?" Pay attention to what you find.

Breathing is a marvellous way of removing toxins from the body. My own experience has taught me that sitting still and breathing deeply after an enjoyable (and indulgent) night out has helped me to feel a lot less cloudy headed. So pay attention to how you feel when you breathe a certain way. Use your breath to enhance your life.

Anatomically, remember that your ribs (which hold your lungs) are primarily behind you. See if you can breathe into your back and be aware of your response.

WHAT YOU NEED

Yourself and an even floor are the essentials. A yoga mat is helpful, but by no means indispensable. Just make sure that the mat, rug or towel you have chosen stops your legs from slipping, to prevent unexpected split postures.

As for clothes, wear anything you find comfortable. I recommend a warm room and your underwear, since this is comfortable and allows you to watch your body move.

Listen to your body. It will tell you when you prefer to practise, but a good tip is that an empty stomach is less distracting than a full one.

Apart from these guidelines, you are your own boss. If spending lots of money helps to inspire you to practise then spend away, but remember – all you need is you and the floor.

A SERIOUS NOTE ON SAFETY

This book is an outline of instructions. It is not a one-to-one personal training session. It cannot watch you or tell you when you are going too far, not working hard enough or using the wrong set of muscles. Only you can do this. Only you can check to see if the weight of your body is in your hips, not your lower back; if your knee is in line with your big toe and hip; if the pain you are feeling is that of muscle burn or a sharp pain that comes from a ligament strain or tear. Take responsibility for yourself; it is much more empowering in the long run. Take your time: feel. There are plenty of reminders along the way.

below These close-ups of parts of the body need to be joined together in order to see the bigger picture, then we are able to see how one thing can relate to another.

core strength

Strength in the centre of the body enables all the other parts to operate more easily. Learn how it feels to pull in the muscles of the abdomen. Combine this with flexibility in the hips and strength in the back, and you are on your way back to the centre of your body.

FLEXIBILITY OR STRENGTH

below Flexibility and strength go inextricably together. As bent, twisted and constricted as some of these postures may appear, the purpose is to help your body find its natural line and balance. Strong joints are the most supple, and strong muscles are the most elastic.

Try not to think of flexibility and strength as two quite separate concepts, or as an "either/or" option. The body is extremely clever so pay attention to what it is telling you.

Watch a young child standing, sitting and moving about freely and you will quickly recognize how far most adults have travelled from paying attention to their own bodies' guidance. Often, we are not even aware that we are setting an insidious pattern until it has become completely ingrained and we are suffering the effects of poor posture, tension and stress.

Flexibility comes from strength and the reason for this is simple. A joint sits between opposing muscles like a see-saw with the tight muscle holding the see-saw down. To create flexibility in a joint you must use the strength of the opposing muscle to stretch its partner.

The first reason why you have these problems is because the body has adapted itself to move, sit and hold itself in the way you have chosen (not how it may have told you to). So now it is the perfect manifestation of who and how you are. This is most obviously illustrated by the way we compensate for a physical injury, but it is actually also happening in ordinary, everyday life. The second reason is that the body tends to open up only when it truly feels safe to do so.

RELEASING THE BODY

There are three common methods of making the body feel safe and of releasing the tightness that hides a weakness. First, you can just collapse and relax, letting everything go, only to find precisely the same tensions and tightness return once you stop relaxing and re-adopt your habitual patterns and methods of movement. Second, you can have the tensions massaged, or manipulated, into letting go, but, once again, your habitual methods and patterns of movement will encourage the original tension back into your body. You could, however, create balance between your muscles, and since balance is most definitely safe, the body – your body – is more likely to open up and let go, altering your habitual patterns and methods of moving for the better. Only when a weakness is strengthened to balance a tense strength will the tension in the body be resolved.

As you practise, be aware of the imbalances in your body; learn to recognize them in everyday life so your work on the mat carries on all day, every day, changing your body from slouch to sleek. Until you balance the "see-saw" in everyday movement the imbalance will remain.

Try to be patient. Be honest about your weakness, then take time to strengthen it until your body makes it clear to you that the weakness is ready to let go.

GRAVITY – USE THE FLOOR

What is the one thing that helps you stay on this planet? It is the same thing that shrinks us during the day and without which we would float away. Gravity beats us down and also provides us with all that we need to find a magical lift. Remember Isaac Newton: for every action there is an equal and opposite reaction. To find this lift up, against gravity's pull, all you need is a body and a floor.

No matter what part of your body is touching the floor or chair, you can find the lift up simply by pushing down a little. After all, we are designed with a foot that has natural balance owing to its arch and a spine that has curves to give us more spring. Gymnasts, yogis, dancers and athletes alike all perform feats that seem to defy gravity because they have found this lift.

More importantly than the ability to perform great feats, this lift shows us that you do not have to suffer under the seeming oppression of the weight of gravity. After all, if you measure yourself in the morning and again that evening there will be evidence that you have shrunk a little in between. This difference between the freedom and length of our spine before and after our day is a major reason why we get tired. The stress of gravity seems against us.

PUSH DOWN TO LIFT UP

But how can levitation be achieved when gravity is so essential to all our lives? Well push down a little. Try and find where gravity is affecting your body, where the weak points are.

Try slouching when you sit and then pushing your bottom down on the seat. Stay there pushing and slouching until you feel the need to let go and you will find that there is a natural lift that accompanies the letting go. You will now feel upright and in line with gravity, not fighting against it. Try the same technique but standing this time and if the feeling remains elusive stay with the pushing and slowly let go with as much awareness as you can muster.

Feel this lift and as it becomes familiar let your actions and movements become filled and dictated by it; never slouching or stooping, always feeling a light long spine being filled with a lift. If you take away the stress and energy used in struggling every day against gravity, you can see how much easier living would be.

So we can forget about the long fight with gravity, and instead give in and use it to our advantage. Regardless of whether you use this to leap like a gazelle, stand on one hand or levitate, it will mean that as you age – the one thing you cannot avoid – you will not stoop, bow or give in to the pull of gravity. You will grow old gracefully.

below You don't have to know about Newtonian mechanics to understand how to use gravity to give you a lift up. See how the hand and the foot both have natural arches, which act like springs pushing up against gravity. Try simply pushing them down and waiting to feel a natural lift in reply.

PULLING THE STOMACH IN

The image of the body beautiful is constantly with us, whether in the media, with new looks of the rich and famous or in adverts for new and miraculous supplements or exercise fads. What is this image? Well it tends to have toned hips and legs with a pert bottom, a strong stomach and an

open chest. Only the genetically gifted or determined fitness freaks seem to embody this ideal, and yet this is in fact how everyone is designed. We all have bigger muscles in our legs than our arms because nature intended us to use our legs as our means of transport. Around our middles are muscles in a similar shape to a girdle that hold our internal organs in the right place. Along our spines are muscles similar to struts that can hold the spine long. In the middle of our body we have a big hinge, the hips, surrounded and protected by big muscles (thighs, buttocks, hamstrings), which help us move around it.

So if we move using our hips as a hinge and our legs as support they will be fitter and toned. If we then hold ourselves upright using our "girdle" and maintain a long spine with our "struts" we will then not tend to let our stomachs bulge and our shoulders collapse.

Through rediscovering how our body is meant to move by feeling it from inside, the perfect body is achievable, and your own ideal body will emerge. You have to put time and intelligence into regular practice of course, but this can include walking, bending, playing games, entertaining and household chores, for they all involve you moving, and it is in this moving you can exercise, and enjoy discovering your body. Discovery does not have to be limited to set practice times for it is in the moments off the mat, sitting at your desk or doing the washing-up, that you understand the satisfaction of living correctly through your body.

Perhaps most interestingly, when you do start to move as you are meant to, your preconceptions of what you should look like fall away. An infinitely more satisfying feeling replaces them, that of a feeling of being at home within your own skin.

left To come out of the ape pose, really suck your stomach up and into your ribs. The position of the hips in relation to the spine is the reason we can walk tall. The more we can make our spine feel that it extends out of our hips, the more we will feel upright and evolved.

ape or man

Poor habits, sitting at a desk, leaning and slouching, can all result in standing incorrectly, putting strain on parts of the body. With poor posture, the weight of the world really does rest on your shoulders and will eventually push you into the ground.

1 Our bodies are remarkably similar to those of apes – we share similarly proportioned limbs and joints – and yet our posture is markedly different. Part of this is due to the way we use our spine, in particular our lower spine. Through playing at copying the stance of an ape we can understand how we became upright and perhaps more importantly what muscles are responsible for this step up in evolution.

To copy the ape stance, let your legs be slightly wider than hip-width as this will give your hips some space to move through, and let your arms hang down, opening your back. Give yourself permission to play and be silly; after all you will look ridiculous sticking your bottom out and letting your arms hang down, so you might as well have fun while you do it. To get back to an upright stance first try squeezing your buttocks and letting your hips come forwards. The feeling is almost as if the muscles of your bottom are pushing you forward (try not to slouch as you slowly stand upright). Repeat this as many times as you need to, until you begin to realize how important your bottom is.

2 The variations on upright vary with perception and reality, especially when our habitual patterns constantly reaffirm themselves in our posture. Take this slouch as an example. The weight of the world is beginning to fall off the rounded shoulders, making life uncomfortable for both the shoulders and the world that sits on them.

3 Look, too, at the slump here, in which the weight of the world sits happily on the shoulders but all the pressure falls to the middle, which begins to bulge as a result. Practise coming in and out of ape until you begin to feel the hinging of your hips forwards and backwards, since this is the reason we can walk tall, without bulges.

abdomen tuck

Most of the stomach exercises we are used to performing seem to make the abdomen bulge out, but the core muscles of the body are made active by pulling in. Therefore, begin by lying flat on the floor on your front.

1 Rest your forehead on your hands and feel the weight of your body on the floor. Feel the front ribs and pelvis pressing into it. You are going to try to pull your stomach up off the floor, keeping your ribs and pelvis down.

2 Begin by simply pulling the tummy up and lowering it down. How high can you pull your stomach up from the floor? Can you feel the lower spine lengthen? Have you created a gap underneath your body? When you feel confident with this, move on.

3 Keep the lower ribs firmly grounded on the floor and your hip bones and pubic bone flat on the floor. Now pull your tummy in as high as you can. Feel the lower spine lengthen and push your legs straight – so straight that you feel your toes spread.

▶ **4** Push your left hip and upper thigh up by squeezing the buttock and lifting your left foot off the floor. Is your tummy still in? Repeat, inhaling alternate legs up, exhaling them down. Can you begin to feel that the tummy can remain in, while the lower spine is kept long, even when you move your legs? Try to gain control of those pulling-in muscles as your limbs are moving.

Lengthen the raised leg from the thigh, as opposed to lifting by squeezing the buttocks. This exercise has the advantages of pulling your tummy in and of relieving tension from the front of your hips – a major cause of lower back pain. It can also lift the buttocks and add shape in quite a short time. With this, and all the exercises in this book, be sure to feel the exercise, not just in your head but throughout your body, so that the sensations make sense.

stomach curl

The pubic lift starts in the stomach. It is very easy just to squeeze your bottom to tuck in your tailbone, which provides the same action. Pay attention to the feeling of the correct action – allowing pressure to be equally distributed throughout the body will relieve problems.

1 Sit with the soles of your feet on the floor and your knees in the air. Sit up as high as you can, pushing your sitting bones down into the floor. Cup your hands on your knees, so as not to use your arm strength to interfere with the exercise.

2 As you roll back, point your toes into the floor and feel your thighs work and lengthen and your knees push down towards the floor. As you come up, pull your heels towards your buttocks. The hamstrings and deep abdomen will engage to pull you up.

3 Look down at your stomach and pubic bone so you can see how you are moving. Using both hands, grab hold of your lower ribs and lift them up. Now suck in your stomach and all the muscles that connect from the pubic bone all the way up the front of the body.

4 As you roll backwards, keep lifting your ribs. You will find that your stomach will pull in as before, but now also up into your rib cage, making it possible to feel a lift in the body as you roll down. Try to detect the origin of the movement in the groin. The fact that the tummy pulls in so hard gives a feeling that the pubic bone is lifted, which in turn tucks the spine between the buttocks and rolls you down.

incorrect If you simply lean back, rather than roll back, the tummy will bulge. If the arms lengthen before the pubic bone has rolled up, you will know that you have simply leaned back from your chest. This will most probably be accompanied by your abdomen pushing out. The pressure here is in your lower back, not spread evenly in the body, and will cause you problems and pain eventually.

elbow lift

In this exercise extend through your legs to your feet, feeling the work in the thighs. Push your chest high off the floor so you can feel the space between your shoulder blades. This will strengthen your stomach muscles, and train them to hold your insides in.

1 Lie on your front and tuck your toes under your heels. Place your hands together, thumbs on your sternum, tucking your elbows in towards your ribs and then push yourself up to balance on your elbows and toes.

2 Lift your pubic bone into your stomach, as in the stomach curl. Practise pulling your abdomen in and up without sticking your bottom out, as that will disengage the stomach muscles, which is the part of you that this exercise is designed for.

alternative If you find this too tricky, rest your knees on the floor, but make sure you really pull your pubic bone up into your stomach and lengthen the lower spine, or the hip flexors will get a good workout and nothing more.

incorrect This shows the classic collapse that usually happens when people try this exercise for the first time. The extremities, especially the toes, take the weight of the body and the lower spine collapses and will soon begin to feel the strain.

HIP FLEXORS

In medical circles, hip flexors are known as iliopsoas. They are very powerful muscles and especially easy to overuse. You will have noticed in the Abdomen Tuck how difficult it was to lift the leg while pushing the hip down. This is caused by tight hip flexors. When they become

permanently tight, the hip bones are constantly being pulled down, emphasizing a lumbar curve in the spine. This leads to a tight lower back and disengages and weakens the abdominal muscles. For this reason, you may feel most tummy exercises in the legs, particularly in the tops of the thighs. However, the more you work on pulling your tummy in and lifting your pubic bone, the more you will feel the abdomen engage, not just during exercises for the stomach but in all your postures. This is the beginning of finding a lift inside you. Don't give in to gravity: be part of it.

LOOSENING THE HIPS

The hips are probably the most important set of hinges in the human body. Protected and worked by the largest group of muscles in the body, they set us apart from all other animals by giving us the ability to move around and function completely upright. The great versatility of the hip joint means that we can lunge forwards (Forward Bend), backwards (Back Bend) and perform any number of combinations of movements involving our legs.

In order to provide independence of leg from torso, there must be a certain level of openness and flexibility within the hips. Constriction limits both the range of movement and the flow of energy. First, let's find out how to improve the flexibility of the hips.

A NOTE FOR WOMEN

Wearing high heels tilts the pelvis forwards, bringing a strong contraction of the hip flexors and a pronounced arch to the lower spine. This not only weakens the lower abdomen and tightens the lower spine, but can also severely limit the range of motion within the hips.

left To feel like your body is truly fluid and free, learn to extend your limbs and make space between them and your body. Open the space at the back of your neck, between shoulders and ears, lift your tummy to help you extend your legs, and then all postures will begin to make more sense.

diamond curl

This exercise stretches the lower back and loosens the hips. However, if you are doing it properly and rolling from the public bone, you will feel the main stretch in the muscles of your legs, especially the hamstrings, which stretch down the back of the thigh.

1 Sit on the floor, as you did for the Stomach Curl, but with your legs in a diamond shape. Place your hands firmly on your knees, pushing them down towards the floor. Feel the hip girdle move firmly forwards and backwards as you roll from the pubic bone.

2 As you roll back, don't be afraid of using your hands. Grab hold of your knees firmly if you need to. Remember to roll your pelvis and feel the movement of your hips between your legs. No matter how flexible you are, there is always room for improvement.

3 Really lean forwards, using your hips as a hinge, and you will feel a tug in your hamstrings, the backs of your legs and the inner thighs, as you roll the hips up and over your legs.

incorrect Leading with your head rather than moving your hips forwards will not exercise your lower back or stretch your leg muscles. Shift your awareness away from your head, which is so accustomed to leading most of the time.

assembly position

Remember sitting cross-legged at school? This exercise is very good for increasing flexibility in the hip joints and the elasticity of the spine. It also helps to stretch and strengthen the buttocks. Try to repeat this sequence at least twice a day and you will notice the difference very quickly.

1 Sit cross-legged. Keep tall, pushing your sitting bones down into the floor to find a lift up inside your abdomen. Place your hands on your knees and lower the shoulders, keeping the neck, shoulders and jaw relaxed.

2 The important step now is to hinge forwards and over your legs from your hips, not by simply collapsing your spine. Lean forwards and pull your stomach in tight. You should feel as though you are pushing your sitting bones backwards into the floor.

3 Lie on your back and bring your knees up into your chest in the Baby position. Begin by rolling your knees, one hand on each, down into your chest. As you do this, keep your bottom, sacrum and tailbone on the floor. If you can do this, you will find that the stretch enters your lower spine and buttocks, just where it should be. Keep the work close to the joint, in the flesh, not the bone.

When you find that the lower spine has released a little, grab hold of your heels by taking your arms inside your legs, then slowly pull your knees down to the floor. You should again play the game of keeping your lower back and top buttocks on the floor.

advanced If that was easy for you, try this. Place the ankles on the opposite knees, crossing the shins, and lean forwards from the hips as before. If possible, place one shin directly upon the other. If this is very comfortable, then draw the knees together until the knees sit inside the shins. The more you lean the greater the stretch you will feel in the top of the thighs.

When you have finished lengthening over both legs and opening both hips, roll onto your back and assume the Baby position to complete the stretch.

pubic lift

The hip flexors dominate your range of movement in this exercise, by using the strength in your abdomen, and bringing you a greater tilt into or openness of the front of the hips. Don't confuse this lift with tucking in your sacrum, pay attention to lengthening your lower spine.

1 Begin in a kneeling position, knees placed directly under your hips. The feeling you are after here is one of lifting your pubic bone with your stomach muscles. Do not be afraid to grab, poke or hold on to bits of you to help feel and discover how your body works.

It is easy just to squeeze your buttocks and tuck your tail under. However, there is another way that will show you the relationship between your tummy and your lower spine. Pull your stomach in.

2 Pull your abdominal muscles in and up as hard as you can, so that your pubic bone is pulled up between your legs. Repeat this in blocks of up to 21 repetitions. You may inhale as you pull your stomach in and up, as this can activate the stomach deeper, so lifting the pubic bone higher. However, if you find it easier to use the out breath to lift and the in breath to lower, then do so.

incorrect Poking your chest out and leaning back slightly will leave your hips in the same position without moving your pelvis. Instead, try to pull your tummy in, especially above your pubic bone. If you cannot find this feeling then go back to pulling in and up. Keep practising and it will appear.

THE BACK – IT'S BEHIND YOU

Your back is beautiful. It is the most amazing construction: 32 pillars stacked perfectly together, which not only hold your head high but also protect the spinal cord, allowing you to move your front so easily.

If we use our backs properly, we find we hinge in the right places. We hang our arms from our shoulders so that no tension is felt in the neck; we move with our backs so that our limbs are drawn into us, in a way that is centred, graceful and effortless. The back – our unseen part – can be our ultimate strength.

The problem is that our eyes point forwards and our backs are behind us. Consequently, we do not care for the one thing that we rely on – our backs. Since our backs are out of sight, they become out of mind to the extent that we cannot feel them; and if we cannot feel them, how can we be aware of changing or using them? The two main tools that you require to "find" your back are patience and practice.

GETTING BACK TO BASICS

Let's take a look at some games. First, can you lift your arms without using your neck muscles or the muscles that lie at the top of your chest or back? Most of us use the muscles at the top of the body, outside our core, to lift, pull, push or stabilize, whereas the body – which is very clever – has some muscles directly between the shoulder blades that can pull the shoulder blades down the back, so lifting the arms. What is the importance of this? Well, if you get neck ache, or even a headache, it is usually as a result of tension in the upper back and neck. Doesn't it make sense then that if there is no tension there, there will also be no pain? This simple exercise is one of the most fundamental steps in re-educating your body about where it stores its stress. The less stress that is stored around the head, the less stress is felt.

Raise your arms just above your head, so that your upper arms and body form a "Y" shape. Hold them there. Gradually your shoulders will open as the back gains strength, so less and less tension is felt in the top of the body. This will yield many benefits to your practice. Remember, the main reason behind all these exercises is to raise your awareness of your body, so try them out with the assurance that there is a purpose to them.

left Stand up straight and place your hands just above your head, with the arms active and outstretched. Keep your elbows bent and out to the sides. As you breathe regularly, feel your shoulders opening and the tension draining away from your upper body.

ape back

Lots of yoga postures were inspired by animals. This one mimics the ape. Copy the animal by leaning forwards and hanging your arms from your shoulder sockets as if your knuckles are about to drag on the floor. This will open your back and also relieve tension around the shoulders.

1 Let your body hang loose and you will feel all the weight in your legs from your hips to your bent knees. Your body should feel strong and open. But do not drop your chest, as this will pull all the weight of your head and upper body into your lower back muscles.

2 This profile captures the "dangle" aspect of the "ape man" pose. The chest is not drooping, so all the weight of the upper body is evenly distributed between all the back muscles that run along the spine and the legs and hips.

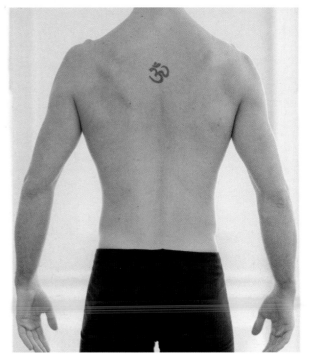

3 To get to the "man" part of this ape game is simple. Pull your tummy in and up hard so that this action will pull you into an upright posture. The challenge is to maintain that open feeling in between your shoulder blades and all the way down to your hands.

4 There is no squeezing or scrunching of shoulders to accompany the in and up tummy from "ape" to "man". In fact, the back hinges up in one long line from the hips without a bend, lean or slouch.

drop the chest and feel the lift

To lift the chest, you find the abdomen caves in and the back arches. However, there is another way. Let's return to training the abdomen. This exercise also helps to strengthen the muscles around the spine and relieves tension and aches in the back.

1 Lie on your front with your pubic bone and bottom ribs on the floor, lengthening the lower spine and engaging muscles of the stomach. Let your shoulder blades broaden and lift your elbows off the ground continuing to roll the shoulder blades down your back. Learn to recognize the feeling of an open chest and open back.

2 Now lengthen the back of your neck and continue to draw the shoulder blades down (you won't move much). The harder you contract the more the upper chest will lift. Keep your ribs and pubic bone down while lifting the stomach up. Simply inhale and try to lift the chest from the back and exhale, letting yourself down slowly.

3 Try to hold yourself up by the muscles that line the spine in between your shoulder blades and raise your legs alternately. Keep your tummy off the floor and raise the arms to the level of the body, but no more, palms uppermost.

arm lift

You can do this exercise standing up or sitting down, but, whichever you choose, it is worth checking yourself visually by watching the movement in a mirror. This will help you identify what you are feeling and allow you to take control of the way you move.

1 Begin with one arm and place the tip of the forefinger on your other hand on the end of your collar bone. Now simply lift your arm up until you find you are lifting your finger. Try to feel the shoulder blade drop down as you lift your arm.

When you have got the idea single armed, try with both arms, but watch and stop when either the top of the chest or the neck begins to become involved.

2 Relax your neck and shoulder muscles as you lift your arm. Looking in the mirror, notice the space that appears between your head and shoulder as you lift your arm. As you lower it, relax your neck and shoulder again and feel the tension disappear. Practise, raising the other arm in exactly the same way.

incorrect If your finger becomes squashed between the neck and shoulder, then you are not doing it correctly. In this picture the shoulder blades have lifted, and space is not being created in the armpit. Don't cheat, as this will stop you from feeling – the only way you will gain control and change the way you move.

basic back bend

Now you have opened up the front of your hips, your lower spine should have lengthened down between the buttocks. All you need to do now is lengthen the rest of the spine on top of the hips and you will find yourself in a Back Bend without having bent your back.

1 Begin as you did in the Pubic Lift, kneeling down with your knees placed directly under your hips. Rest your hands on your hips.

2 Suck in your stomach muscles to lift the pubic bone up and through your thighs while you lift and extend your spine. This should keep your tummy tight and trim, and when you recognize that feeling, you can be sure that the spine is protected and long.

▶ **3** Place both hands on your upper chest and push your hands up with your body. Keep the back of your neck long. Do not stop the lift in your tummy and pubic bone. The chest should feel as though it is moving forwards and upwards, rather than downwards and backwards. If you feel pressure or discomfort in your lower spine or it feels as if your lower back is doing all the work, go back to opening up the front of your hips and thighs, as this is still limiting the extension of your lower back.

incorrect If you do not lift your pubic bone and simply lean backwards you will find that the back will bend a lot but you will only move backwards a little.

alternative If you find the Back Bend difficult, use your hands. Push your thumbs into your sacrum to help hinge the hips up and use your arms to help brace the back out long from the hips. If you feel pain or work in your lower spine, go back to practising Pubic Lifts.

BACK TO FRONT

How can you tell what's going on behind you? Can you feel when your back is long? Without the aid of some friendly angled mirrors it is almost impossible to see your back. However, you do have the advantage of having a perfectly good mirror that is always in view, called your stomach. When you stand or sit, watch how your front behaves; as these three examples show, it will help you see what is going on behind you.

1 ARCHING SPINE

First there is the time when your stomach sticks out, especially the portion below your navel. Try it out, let your stomach relax forwards and you will feel your lower back begin to arch (see the illustration below).

This is for the simple reason that your stomach is pulling it forwards, and if the spine remains in this pulled position for too long you will feel an ache in your lower spine. The obvious solution to this is to pull your tummy

back in, which will in turn allow the spine to move back and your weight to be carried evenly between the front and the back.

2 HIGH CHEST

Next, try pushing your ribs forwards. A squeezing together of the shoulder blades normally accompanies this projection of your rib cage, so try that as well if you wish. If you now pull your shoulder blades down you will feel a collapsing sensation in your spine. This is due the middle area now being compressed. Picture 2 showing the back view shows this pronounced dip, which is rather worrying when you consider that your kidneys are being compressed. To bring yourself back into line, place your hands on your ribs and pull your ribs away from your hands. Combine this action with allowing your chest to soften while keeping your upper back long to iron out that middle back dip.

3 HIP BALANCE

You can often see on people with a pronounced hip imbalance that one side of the waist is longer than the other. When this is the case you can guarantee that one side of the spine is longer than the other, and probably twisting, which can lead to back and hip problems. To get your hip bones even, push the sitting bone on the raised side down whilst keeping that side of the waist long. Sitting on the floor, or on your heels, is probably one of the best positions to do this since the floor will bring awareness to your sitting bones.

Keep an eye on these three principals as you practise and you will be able to know how to see when your hips are balanced and your spine is long.

1 back and front If your tummy pushes out and your hips rock forwards, then you know that there is a lumbar curve in your back. This is how so many lower back problems begin. Lengthen the abdomen to lengthen the spine and relieve the pressure caused by this constriction.

balancing the spine

These three examples show common ways that the back is misaligned. You might only be alerted to this imbalance of the back by the state of your front. Once you become aware of the pitfalls, a protruding chest, or distended stomach will alet you to more serious problems.

2 front If your chest puffs out and up, then you know you would see a heightened thoracic curve. You need to allow the chest to soften and the tummy to lift.

2 back Imagine that your kidneys are being squeezed by this curve in the lower back, and you will understand that it is worth correcting it. This is what happens when the chest is out.

3 front If one side of your body protrudes. and twists, it is merely mirroring the arc of your spine. You have to find out which of your sitting bones needs to lift, ground it, and then lift it into the rest of the body.

3 back If one side of your waist is longer than the other, as in this picture, then your spine is collapsing or bending to the opposing side. You need to push down the sitting bone to lengthen the waist to pull the spine back into line.

SOLID GROUNDING

Even the most generally perfect bodies have at least one area that needs special attention. If you are reading this bemoaning how much of your body does not work, think about two things. First, your body is already fairly perfect because it has got you this far. Second, the work never stops for anyone; perfection is never achieved.

Be aware of the power of imbalances in the body. Continually repeating an action with an unbalanced shoulder or hip girdle will guarantee a habitual pattern that will twist and corrupt your body. You will not realize this until your body seems to give out for the smallest and most ridiculous of reasons: "I must have twisted strangely", or, "It happened just as I was getting out of bed."

However, the good news is that there are many bodies that have gone from being round-shouldered, humped, arched and twisted to long, open, lithe and strong. You will need to be constantly vigilant and aware, but with this will come the joy of truly knowing your own body, of truly knowing yourself.

It is recommended that you find an excellent physiotherapist, as he or she will aid your awareness of where you are habitually tight or soft. He or she will recommend exercises, probably quite similar to the ones in this book, which you must practise regularly. Simply having a diagnosis and a list of exercises is not enough; if you do not put these exercises into practice, you will not change.

KEEP CHANGING

Change the way you use your muscles, for they are the main reason why you are pulled out of shape. Your body is not set in stone. The only limit to change is you.

Do not be scared of treating your body to a session at the physiotherapist or masseur/se to loosen your muscles. If you invest in your body, it should run well for a lot longer: you do that for your car, after all. By taking your body to a specialist in bodies – whether a doctor, a physiotherapist, or a masseur/se – you can find out how to take an interest in your speciality. But whatever their advice, make sure that it makes sense in your body.

Take pride in being special. You have the best reason to become exceptional: to make your weakness your strength. If you can be brave enough to find, accept, know and love your weaknesses, you will find an inspiration that could unlock far more than the balancing of your hips.

left Standing on one leg, wearing high-heeled shoes, slouching or sitting badly when you are working: all these things will contribute to poor posture. In the long run this may cause scoliosis, or curvature of the spine. It is never too late to take control of your habits, and your body.

flat feet – flat feeling

If your arches have collapsed then you will not be leaping around with a spring in your step.
It is crucial to get your foundations correct, then you will have a stable support structure for the
rest of your body.

correct The ankle is in the middle of the foot with the toes spreading the weight of the body evenly across the entire ball and heel of the foot. When the foot looks like this, there is a natural spring to it, as opposed to flat and floor bound. To find this balance and placement of the ankle on the foot, have a look at the Jimmy Choo posture.

incorrect Look how the ankle bone is falling away from the centre of the foot. This collapse not only brings about a collapsed arch – flat feet – but also gradually pulls the big toe towards the outside of the foot. This will eventually affect the inside of the knee – knock knees – and then affect the hip as it travels up the leg.

correct Compare the picture on the right with this and you will see the muscles in this foot holding up the arch and the ankle in the middle of the foot. The arch is there in most of us, but if it is not, in most cases it just requires us to condition the muscles of the foot for the arch to appear.

incorrect Look how little gap there is between the floor and the foot. In such little space, it is hard to feel a lift or bounce. The lift has to start where your body is in contact with the floor, and if the foot has collapsed, there will not be much lift. Try doing the Jimmy Choo exercises whenever you can to correct this condition.

ANKLES, KNEES AND HIPS

Let's begin with the ankles. Get a mirror and get honest. Have a good look. Which ankle corresponds to which picture?

You will probably find that one ankle lies differently from the other. When you stand, your feet probably do not point forwards at the same angle. This imbalance is repeated each time you step, walk or run, winding its way up through your knee to your hip and into your spine.

To correct the imbalance, let's use the mirror, your feet and some of your concentration.

KNEES

Whether you are bow-legged or knock-kneed, by paying attention to the relationship between your ankles and your hips you can literally lengthen your legs. When you maintain the lift in your

arches, your ankles will not want to collapse. Down Dog is a perfect posture in which to work on knees and ankles. After all, you can look at them from the best position. Practise rolling your ankles and playing with the feet, until you feel the relationship between your hips and your heels.

HIPS: LEARN TO BE HERE

When someone claims that one of their legs is longer than the other, it is almost always actually the case that they are holding one of their hips higher than the other. Do you cross one leg in preference to the other? Do you stand with your weight on one hip? These habits mirror and reinforce an existing imbalance. This is not to say that you must sit or stand properly on both sitting bones or feet for the rest of your days, only that you need to become aware of your body.

Go back to feeling. Are your hip bones even? Go back to the hip opening sequence at the beginning of the book.

THE JIMMY CHOO

This exercise is named after the designer of beautiful, but unfeasibly high-heeled shoes. It is designed to help you overcome fallen arches. Simply lift and lower your heels, keeping everything in line – it's harder than it sounds – and your feet should wake up. You can use something to help you balance, but if possible keep your hands on your hips and see if you can feel a lift in your tummy as you raise and lower yourself. This will bring your awareness to the connection between your feet and you.

left Down Dog is the best posture to examine the relationship between your feet, ankles and knees because you are looking straight at them. Play inside this posture. Try collapsing your ankles followed by bringing them into the middle of the foot. As you do, feel your knees move in and out of line and maybe even become aware of the use of the muscles in your groin. It is up to you to make time within this and all postures to learn how best your body works.

the Jimmy Choo

It really doesn't matter if you can't get your heels as high as is shown in the picture on the left. Push the balls of the big toes down and feel the lift of the heels up. As long as you feel this, you are heading in the right direction. With this feeling you will begin to make your foundations firm.

1 Stand with your feet facing forwards directly underneath your hips, everything perfectly parallel. Lift your heels up tall, on tiptoes (demi-point). Try to lift them directly above the balls of your big toes. Make sure that the ankles do not fall to the left or right and you will find that the feet are stimulated, the arch stretched and strengthened and strong lines formed from the foot through the ankle to the knee and hip.

2 Open your toes and spread them wide to give you a firm base, pressing them down to help you balance. When you have risen up and down on your toes enough to feel familiar with the action, concentrate on going straight up, trying not to lean forwards each time you lift up. Use the wall to help if you need to, but when you lift up directly, you will feel the direct stimulation of the arches of the feet.

3 If your ankles collapse inwards stretch your little toes to keep your ankles in the middle of your body.

4 When your ankles fall out press the ball of your big toe into the floor and stretch your big toe forwards.

5 When both ankles are over the ball of your foot push your ankle forwards to help stimulate your arches.

standing postures

Now you have found where the core strength of your body is centred, it is time to begin your practice with the standing postures. Some of these may be a challenge to your body, so begin gently and gradually build up, holding the poses for slightly longer periods of time.

STANDING START

By now you should have successfully figured out how to feel and use your core strength. You can hold yourself, warm up your body, move and, most important, feel when your body is working happily. Now it is time to challenge your body with standing postures.

To begin with, the demands made on the body by these postures will feel unnatural. But remember the idea of flow around the body. By using your core strength to hold you up, you begin to use the body as a pump to increase the flow of energy. So you should approach this section in two ways, looking at both individual shapes and postures and how you flow between them.

There are instructions on where you will feel each posture most, but it is important that you really look at the pictures and trust that your brain will make sense of them and interpret them into your body – it might help to use a mirror. Remember, there is no wrong feeling, only you, at that moment. If you look and read carefully you will have more than enough information to decide whether what you are doing is as beneficial as it can be. Bear in mind that you will fully feel a posture only after practice over time.

FLOWING MOVEMENT

The standing postures are designed to flow together. You can take a quick look through the book to see the bigger picture, but just as you are made up of little pieces, so is the sequence. Try to enjoy putting the sequence together, much as you might have enjoyed putting yourself together with your core in the first section.

Do not be scared to stop, play, or notice when something in you begins to feel. If you feel really comfortable, enjoy the feeling of your body working, flowing, not giving in to gravity. When a posture is hard, try the alternative version. When it is easy, stay longer, go deeper, extend further. If you feel discomfort, you should check that your core is working properly and that you are being true to your alignment and flexibility. Do not persist with a posture that is causing you pain, but carefully check the instructions and pictures again. Remember that almost all injuries happen when you are not listening, feeling and being honest.

left Build on your ability to feel and use your core strength as you move on to standing postures. After reading the instructions and looking at the photographs, listen to your own body as you practise the postures.

right Be aware of the flow of energy as you move from one standing posture to another and make use of your core strength to increase that flow. Not only will this be beneficial, it will also make your practice more enjoyable.

lunge

Learn to love this posture. Inside it are myriad possibilities, all held static by the lift in the pubic bone and extensions through the thighs. The back heel in demi-point will stimulate the arch of the foot, which in turn allows you to open the hip. Lift the heel and drive the thigh back.

1 Stand with the feet together, extend forwards and touch the floor beside the feet with your fingertips. Look up, lifting the chest, and stretch one leg out behind you. Push one knee forwards and the other backwards (only one way makes sense) and feel the length between the back of your head and heel.

2 Place your hands on your knee as shown here. Put all your emphasis on lifting your pubic bone, lifting the back heel and opening the hip. The arms are down, but are your shoulder blades down too? This is the easy option, so if your legs are tired or if you want to give your tummy a helping hand, stop at this point.

▶ **3** Prop the shoulder blades to lift your arms and regain the feeling of freedom in the neck and shoulders. You should feel as though the torso is exactly the same as when standing, so the legs are required to hold you elegant and tall. The more power there is in your legs, the more lift and openness you will feel in the hips and body.

◀ **incorrect** The front thigh is lower, so all the weight of the body is being carried at the bottom of the lower back, instead of in the hip and thighs. The bulging tummy mirrors the overarched spine, something guaranteed to create an ache if held for too long. Notice also the back foot. Keep the hip and ankle happy by opening both.

pert buttocked warrior

This posture carries straight on from the Lunge. Lower the arms to shoulder height from the full Lunge, and turn to face the side, rather than the front. This posture will help to open the hips, strengthen the legs and knees and reinforce the core strength that you have built up.

▶ **the full posture** From a Lunge, roll the back heel to the floor and allow the hip to follow. If you keep the front knee and hip in the same place you turn flat and into Pert Buttocked Warrior. The pertness comes from a lift in the pubic bone and a rolling backwards of the thigh muscles. This back view shows you the length of the spine which comes from the lift in the pubic bone, the evenness of the hips and the breadth of the back. Notice that the shoulder blades are down and that the neck is free.

◀ **close-up** Here is a close-up of the buttocks, because you need to really feel how lifting the pubic bone and rolling the thighs backwards affects the hips. Put your hands on your bottom and feel this work. You will also notice that the strength of this posture cannot fail to open even the most stubborn of closed hips. The right angle in the knee can be sacrificed for the sake of good buttocks, since stubborn hips are far more important to feel and open than trying for perfection without knowing where it is.

close-up The back foot is again very important. After it has been stimulated in the Lunge, you should keep a lift in the ankle while pushing the heel and ball of the big toe down. This will allow you to feel the body supported by both legs, rather than just by the front thigh. The more you can activate the muscles of the back leg, the easier it will be to feel the connection between the foot and groin. Try it and ground yourself. Through activating the arch of the back foot you will be able to feel the support of the back leg.

correct Look at the long line from the big toe to the knee to the hip. Notice also how the hips are facing flat to one side. Try to make yourself flat in this posture to benefit your hip flexibility and core strength and for the sake of your knee joint.

incorrect Look at the lines. See the stress on the inside of the front knee and how hard the outside of the shin has to work. The arch of the foot has also diminished. The back hip has rolled forwards so the hip cannot be opening as much.

side lunge

In this posture, the front leg has not changed position since the Lunge; the body has just moved around it. When the muscles work together, you will feel how they hold you long and upright and how the opposing forces of your legs provide balanced stability.

1 From the Warrior, lean the body towards the bent knee. Although the elbow is resting on the knee, the length is maintained along both sides of the waist. The hand on the bottom allows the sitting bone to be pulled backwards, and the knee to be pushed forwards.

2 In a simple Side Lunge the arm is lifted until the bicep reaches the nose. Notice the long line from head to heel, and the breadth to the back. Shoulder blades should be kept down and the back of the leg long. Beginners should stop at this stage of the posture.

close-up Notice how the length in the side of the waist is mirrored by that in the spine. The legs, both pushing forwards and pulling backwards, allow the hip to hinge and become stable at the same time, two opposing forces balancing one another to leave stillness. Remember your stomach: keep it off your thigh.

incorrect A nice try with the arms, but a lot of collapse everywhere else. See how the angle between the thigh and waist is not sharp, meaning that the spine has to bend to take the body over. The weight of the body is therefore being held by little muscles, those of the curved spine.

▶ **3** Raise the left arm above the head, keeping the shoulders relaxed and down. The angle from above demonstrates why this posture feels so good. Look at the line from the back of the head. It feels as though the line grows from the floor and allows the back to broaden and separate. Notice the gap between the arms and ears, meaning that tension is held away from the head.

thigh lunge

From the Side Lunge, turn the body to face the front foot. Body weight should be distributed equally between the front and back leg. It is called the Knee Trembler, because the weight of the body is directly over the front thigh and when this thigh gets tired the knee begins to tremble.

1 Keeping the back heel flat on the floor forces you to feel your inner thigh and back leg. Even though your hands and arms are helping to support your torso, keep your tummy up and in. Try not to collapse and stick your bottom out. Beginners can stop here.

2 Take your arms back like a bird, but spread your wings – your shoulder blades – to open your back. Remember that you are never trying to constrict the body, so squeezing your shoulder blades together to "fly" your arms back simply draws tension to your neck.

close-up This back view explains the essence of the posture. The length in the back must mean that the front of the body is long as well. Lean forward from the root of the back heel, but always keep your body free and let it hinge from the front knee and hips.

incorrect The collapse in the upper back means there is even more weight in the lower spine. If your back is feeling the weight, lift your chest and pull your tummy in until your thighs begin to burn gently. Notice how the shoulders are around the ears. Drop your shoulders and extend your neck. Remember the length from your head to your heel.

▶ **3** Raise the arms over the head. Notice that the neck is long, the shoulder blades are low, so again there is no tension in the neck. Notice how the tummy is drawn in and up, helping to maintain the length of the lower spine. Notice, too, the long, straight line through the body. Enjoy separating the knees – one forwards, the other back – and using your back to stabilize yourself. Here's a quick challenge. Can you use your tummy so that you feel buoyant?

dog split

This posture – a cross between Down Dog and the splits – is really quite tricky. My advice is just to go ahead and do the posture. Make sure that you stretch from your back heel to your top toes. In fact, once you're there, it is actually quite fun.

1 After the Thigh Lunge, place your hands on the floor and straighten your leg. Do not blindly push your knee straight, but push your heel down and lift your bottom up. Create some space and some lift off the floor. A quick challenge. Can you lift your leg up between your hands?

2 This is how the Dog Split is most often performed. The leg is lifted back until it makes a long line from wrist to toes. To lift the leg, squeeze your bottom and lengthen your hip. Try looking at your ankle over the bottom foot. Is there a line all the way from your big toe, ankle, knee and hip bone? Beginners, stop at this point.

incorrect This version of the posture is a common mistake. Inflexibility in the chest means that it is hard to keep the shoulders open and arms correctly positioned. A desire to lift the back leg high results in a lifted hip and an inability to detect whether the back leg is straight. The head is up, so welcoming neck tension, and the back heel is down, adding to the collapse.

▶ 3 Feel the floor under your hands and push all the way from your wrists to your toes. Keep your shoulders braced, even and away from your ears. Your hips should be even and your ribs slightly contracted.

◀ advanced You should not attempt this advanced version unless you can already do the splits. If you can, bounce the back foot forwards, root your heel and extend as much as you can through the front hip. Push your bottom up with your thigh (not with your arms, as this tends to lead to constriction), and your abdomen can help. You can use your head and a relaxed neck as a weight to pull the leg up.

press up

This posture's very mechanical nature makes it a constant challenge. Sometimes known as the Staff pose, the body is held long by the torso muscles and, primarily in this posture, the back. If your shoulder blades pop up away from your ribs, try and perfect the easy version.

1 From the Dog Split, bring yourself to this position, pushing your chest high off the floor and lifting your pubic bone up into your abdomen. This will hold you up and away from the floor. To lower yourself, just bend your elbows, nothing else.

2 As you lower your body by bending the elbows, notice that the shoulder blades have not lifted and the chest is still lifted off the floor. Feel this posture in your tummy and back, not your shoulders and chest. If you are just beginning, keep your knees on the floor.

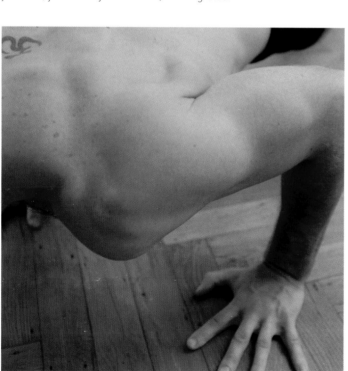

close-up Your back is your strength in this posture. Tuck your shoulder blades down and away from each other to activate your back. Look at the shoulder and the muscle that leads to the neck; there is very little tension in there.

incorrect This is a case of being head bound – when you move your head you think that all of you has moved. People think that the most important part of this posture is to get down and so sacrifice all integrity to get there: collapsed shoulders, chest taking the weight, flaring elbows which detach the arms from any back strength, and a soggy middle.

▶ **3** The arms go no deeper than in this illustration, keeping the shoulders in line with the elbows. Any lower and the chest will constrict and the integrity of your shoulder stability will be compromised. This posture should have no constriction anywhere in the body; in fact, you should actively open your chest, shoulders and back.

up dog

The more you understand the Press Up, the easier and more enjoyable Up Dog will become. Since the work was in the back in the Press Up, you now know just where to lift from to take you into this posture with your chest and shoulders open.

1 The width between the shoulders can be achieved only when the work is inside the back, allowing the chest to open. Notice how the tummy is pulled in and up. The elbows are open, rather than the arm, shoulder and back muscles taking the weight of the body.

2 The thighs are raised off the floor. The shoulders are wide, but follow the "V" shape down the abdomen and you can see that the muscles are pulled in and the pubic bone is lifted up, keeping the thighs off the ground.

▶ 3 See the breadth of the back. The shoulder blades are contained within the back and as wide as they can be to let the head float on top. The redness in the back shows the level of exertion. Use your shoulder blades to lift you and keep your tummy in and legs strong to protect your lower spine.

incorrect The head thrown back without any support means that the cervical (neck) vertebrae are compressed. It is obvious that the chest is not open, and the position of the arms means that there is little hope of involving the back to help lift. Get your wrists beneath your shoulders and push the floor away from you.

incorrect Can you spot the mistakes? The neck is not long, so something is wrong. The chest and shoulders are narrowed forwards, when this posture is meant to open them. The thighs are resting flat on the floor, offering no protection to the lower spine.

down dog

I would prefer to call this posture Bottom Up, for when the sitting bones come up, the lower spine extends and the abdomen lifts up to support the spine. Another name for this pose is Inverted V, and this picture shows the significance of the name.

◄ **1** Down Dog is not easy, as we have a tendency to narrow everything, especially when our legs complain at our bodies being at such a strange angle to them. To flow from Up Dog to here, just pull up the tummy, roll over the toes and push from the wrists to the bottom. Here, the heels do not yet reach the floor, since the Achilles tendons and calves are still rather tight. However, the shoulder blades are wide and away from the head. Keep an eye on your ankles. Is there a line from big toe to hip bones? Are the arches in your feet active?

▶ **2** See how little tension there is inside the back and shoulders. The neck can dangle free and the distance between the shoulders is as wide as possible. This means that any stretch in the chest is not felt at the expense of space and freedom inside the back. Broaden your back, open your shoulder blades and get your shoulders away from your ears. Don't be scared of taking your hands wider than your shoulders, as this will make these actions easier. Use the breadth in the back to open your chest.

close-up Try really spiking your bottom up while pushing your heels down and keeping your stomach muscles lifted. Imagine the sitting bones up near the ceiling. This will keep you light on your hands, long in your spine and free in your hamstrings.

incorrect This demonstrates how not to do this posture. Look at the big curve in the back. This shows that this is more like an inverted "U" than a "V". The neck is long and dangling, but look at the tension in the shoulders. In this position you will find more weight in the wrists, whereas if you look at the close-up, left, you can see that most of the weight in the body should actually be felt in the hips. Don't worry about your heels. Lift your bottom and lengthen your spine.

incorrect This picture looks strong – look at all the activity around the upper back, neck and shoulders. But see how narrow the shoulder girdle is: the distance between the shoulders is minimal. How can this be considered an open posture? Look beyond the muscular appearance and see the constriction.

jump

This Jump is the link between Down Dog and the Forward Bend. Any jump is a challenge until you know you can do it, so this is a lot easier to do when you believe your body will let you. Explode, fly, bounce your bottom in the air – gravity will help with the landing.

1 From Down Dog, bend your knees and push your bottom back and up. This should enable you to feel the leg muscles begin to work. Coil your body up as far away from your hands as possible. Pull in the tummy to hold the spine long and lift the heels high.

2 Push your legs straight up and see how high you can bounce. Lift your heels so your stomach pulls right in. Look at your tummy to see where it's gone. As silly as this may seem, it will help you pull higher off the floor, which in turn introduces you to feeling the lift.

3 Extend right through your hands and arms, since these are the struts that hold up the body when you spring forwards. You are less likely to collapse if you keep your arms strong. From the coiled back position, push your legs straight up, bouncing as high as you can.

incorrect This position says, "I'm scared". Notice the way the back is rounded, the shoulders are rolled in and the body is already heading towards the hands. How can you expect to bounce high from here if the spine is not long, the arms not strong and the thighs not curled to pounce? Try bouncing on the spot before bouncing forwards.

▶ **4** Here is how the feet should meet the floor – as though you have been folded in the middle. Stretch your legs all the way to your toes, so you feel you open up as you jump up. Suck your tummy in so hard that you feel you can stay up there. Aim to land with your feet in between the hands, ready for the Forward Bend on the following page. This position requires strength, balance and flexibility, and when you find them, your body can move and jump just as you imagine it can.

forward bend

On landing from your Jump, you are almost there. Find the hinge in the hips, and then allow both the backs of the legs and the lower back to lengthen from the top point. All you need to do is push your heels down and lift your bottom. It's that simple.

1 A Forward Bend does not require straight legs. Always keep your chest against your thighs to maintain the maximum length in your lower spine. Pull your tummy off your thighs to help you lengthen the lower spine. Then simply push your heels down and push your bottom up. Do not push your knees straight, unless they go easily, as all this will do is take the work away from your upper thighs.

2 Aim for a perfect hinge from your hips no matter how straight you can press your legs. All that pushing your legs backwards will achieve is taking your knee joint beyond the position where it functions most efficiently. Learn to carry the weight of your body in your hips, not in the backs of your knees. Allow your head to relax while you keep lifting your bottom.

incorrect This picture is just to remind you to keep your shoulders away from your head. Allow the back to broaden. It is so easy in your eagerness to bend down low to use the wrong muscles and take the effort and attention away from where it should be – in your hips. Use your legs to go forwards; they are a lot bigger and closer to the hip hinge than your arms.

▶ 3 If you find the Forward Bend easy, take your upper body out of the equation and lift your arms. Can you keep your back broad, your legs long and your chest on your thighs without the aid of your arms? Pull your stomach off your thighs, yet push your head and chest on to your legs. Feel the work in the thighs and abdomen, as this will strengthen the hips and, in turn, deepen the stretch.

incorrect This looks quite flexible and the hands are touching the floor, but look how the spine is bowing to achieve this. Here the hip hinge is wide open. This means the stress is carried in the back and knees, both a little more fragile than the hips and thighs. A Forward Bend does not require straight legs, it requires a movement of the hips towards the thighs.

twisted postures

These are positions to challenge the inside of your body as well as the outside. If you practise them regularly you will feel the benefits in your digestive system and also in your waistline, proving that true beauty starts from within.

seated twist and prayer

It may take some time to become familiar with the sensation of space in your back, but keep searching for it because when you can apply it to a twist, you'll feel a freedom in your spine that you will want to keep.

◀ **1** Begin by standing upright and place your palms together at shoulder height, but as you do, keep as much distance between your elbows as possible. Keep this space as you bend your knees, sit down and twist, for it will help you to maintain some space between your thighs and tummy and also inside your back.

▶ **2** Think of taking your chest forwards and slightly up and your bottom backwards. Check that there is space between your hands and chest. Breathe into your back, breathe out and twist with your tummy. Keep the back of your neck long and remember that your neck is part of your spine, so that if it droops or twists away from that central line of the twist, you are more likely to injure it. Note how the heels, shins and toes are all kept together as a guide to help keep the hips in line. There should be no constrictions. The back is not designed entirely for the purpose of twisting, and twisting it when it is compressed is just silly.

close-up This angle shows the line of the spine. Take a look at where the twist comes from. The lower spine is long and flat, held safe by the tummy. Follow the line up and just underneath the tattoo where the smaller vertebrae of the thorax begin, the twist begins. Let your chest roll round. Use your breastbone as a guide if you cannot feel the twist. Can you keep the top shoulder blade open and the neck long?

incorrect Here we see a twist and droop. The spine is not extended, there is no twist to be seen and the middle of the back will feel the weight of this position. If you find yourself doing this, drop your bottom down and extend your chest. Remember, you have a long spine, so use its full length, otherwise you will begin to feel the strain.

advanced If you are able to do this Pelican pose, it is a good link into the next posture. Gaze at your foot (the one under your elbow) and curl the heel of your other foot towards your bottom. Keep your knees together, as this will help to maintain some stability in the hips and point that foot before getting ready to drive it back.

revolved lunge

Keep this posture simple and do not try to twist too far as you may end up losing all stability. Instead, concentrate on keeping your hips balanced and your back open and when this feels natural, begin to twist around by trying to move your belly button to face your thigh.

1 Having lifted the leg in the Pelican, drive it back as long as is comfortable while keeping that angle in the front knee. Holding your bottom will help you feel this strange sensation of pushing the knee forwards while pulling the hip backwards.

2 This angle shows you the space between the shoulder blades, which are free of constriction. It also shows the wrist under the shoulder and the bicep rolled forwards, since this helps to open the back and roll the shoulders down away from the ears.

close-up This close-up draws attention to the centre of this posture, because in the hurry to extend one leg back and one forwards, lift an arm and feel the floor with the opposite hand, it is easy to forget that you are revolving and that to do so you need your tummy to hold your centre still. Notice that the chest is open and yet the top arm follows the curl of the shoulder forward and is not just pushing up to the ceiling. Think from the centre out. Don't get distracted by your extremities.

incorrect There is a lovely line down the back but look at that top arm. Note how the back has constricted with the desire to find the ceiling. Follow the line of the top arm into the body and you will see that it passes straight out of the shoulder into thin air. It is not securely in the shoulder joint.

▶ **3** As you begin to twist around, be aware of the space beneath you and don't be tempted to droop and crush it. Just remember that when you pull the opposite ends of a twisted towel, it deepens the twist, so keep your chest up and forwards and your back leg driving backwards to create the effect in your body. Follow the line of the top arm and you will see it is carried directly through the shoulder joint. There is no constriction within the top shoulder blade and both the back and the chest are open. The back leg is extended as long as possible and yet all parts of the body are revolved around the middle. Pay attention to your core strength.

side triangle

When you balance on your side, you naturally think that your arm is supporting you. However, the arm does not need to do much work since its bones provide a solid staff. The side of your body is not so solid, so put your attention to using all the muscles down that side to make it stiff.

1 From the Revolved Lunge, put (or keep) your hand on your bottom, push down hard and lean back a little. Your leg will whip itself back in its desire to straighten. Pushing your legs, and keeping them long, and the stomach strong, will help to hold you up.

2 As a prelude to the advanced posture, try this version. Look at the twist in the middle. It requires all your core muscles – tummy, back and hips – to pull together so that you can push and lift at the same time.

alternative Any pain in the wrist, elbow or shoulder will warrant this amendment. However, just because you are using two hands to balance does not mean you can collapse through your middle. In fact, it means you should work your middle even harder.

incorrect You can lower yourself from the first posture to this and back up again, which is a nice exercise, but to hold this position will do little except help you to strain something. There is no space between head and neck and no sign of a lift against gravity. When people first try this version it is such hard work for them. Then, when they find their middle, they feel so much lighter.

▶ **advanced** This looks tough, but is really quite easy. In Side Triangle, make a big tunnel underneath you by pushing off the floor and sucking the side of your tummy up off the floor. Bend the knee so you can lift your top leg to grab hold of the big toe of the top foot. Then simply push the top leg straight while holding on to it. It may take a little time, but it's not that hard.

triangle

With both feet back on the floor, turn to face the side, and you are in Triangle. This is also a twist which starts in the abdomen and ends in the neck, so practise rolling your body behind you, twisting away from the floor and looking up to the ceiling.

1 Holding the buttock of the front leg with the opposite hand, lift it to begin your descent into Triangle pose. Pay plenty of attention to the length in both sides of your waist. Use the same activation of your side tummy muscles as in the last posture.

2 Keep lifting your bottom up, hinging through your hip, until your hand reaches your shin, ankle or foot. Extend both sides of your body. Pull your tummy in and roll your chest back over your thighs. If you are really tight in the legs, place the hand higher.

incorrect Spot the mistakes. The hand is on the wrong buttock, meaning there is no biofeedback in the hamstring of the other leg, no matter how high she lifts. A curvy spine and tilt forwards means the effect of this posture is handed to the middle and lower back, instead of to the muscles of the hip. Lengthen, don't droop.

the correct alignment This shows you how your body ideally sits in line and over your leg. You may have no one to assist you but you still have the ability to close your front ribs and roll your chest backwards over your leg. This will keep your spine long.

▶ **3** How many triangles can you see? There are only two, but the importance of them explains the posture. The underside of the body is a straight line and both sides of the waist are even, which means the spine is kept long. Thus the flexibility for this posture comes from the muscles in the hips rather than from a bend in the back, as curves do not appear in a triangle. The other triangle – of the legs – shows how great this posture is for opening the hips. The hand is on the opposite sitting bone to help pull the bottom up and keep the hamstring of that front leg as long as possible. Don't be boxed in by this posture. Be a triangle.

revolved triangle

This is a difficult posture and should be approached intelligently. It demands great awareness and stability from your hips, while your core strength maintains a length to your lumbar spine and provides a twist above it. Take it slowly until all the parts work together.

◀ **1** From the Triangle, reverse the hands so the buttock is still being lifted, this time by the arm of the same side. The other arm goes to the shin, the ankle or maybe even the floor. Pull in your tummy well and be prepared to really feel the back of your front leg. Push your heel down and lift your bottom up to extend the front leg long. Keep your front long, as this will mean that the spine is more likely to remain long.

▶ **2** Now try placing the hand further down the leg, aiming for the floor by the little toe of the front foot. Look at the triangles in the posture and at the spine. The strength in the legs means that the hips are more likely to open to allow you deeper over your front leg. Really hold and lift your buttock, as this will help you to lengthen your lower spine and extend your chest forwards. Try to keep your back broad as you roll your chest backwards. Try pushing your sitting bone back into your hand while taking your chest forwards. What happens to your leg?

close-up The revolution of the twist is in the tummy. You can see the proof before you. Keep both sides of your waist long and twist. Then maintain this length by pushing your hand backwards. Give your sitting bone a tug up as you do so.

incorrect The wrong buttock is being held, so when you push your hand backwards the result is a twist in the back rather than more length. Also, how can you extend the front leg when you are lifting the back one? Look at the spine on its gentle curve down to the floor, resulting in a floppy head. The hand on the floor is not important. Take your hand higher if you are inflexible, but keep your spine long and keep your body open.

alternative A helping hand is useful with this tricky posture. The reason for this angle is that it shows how the shoulders and hips should align. When they are aligned, the spine will be in a long line as opposed to bending up or curving down. Watch those front ribs as you twist, as they have a tendency to stick out. Closing them will allow you to feel that the back is long, and eliminate any hollow that may appear in the middle.

balanced postures

So what are the advantages of balancing on one leg? We are bipeds, with two legs and two hips providing our main means of movement, and any imbalance between them affects the whole body. By learning to balance on one foot, feeling your weight evenly on the foot through the ankle, both the knee and the hip are strengthened on that side. If both hips are kept even, then not only can hip imbalances be righted but all the torso and core muscles become involved.

triangle forward bend

After all the work so far, you should really be feeling this in the legs. A Forward Bend is found in the hips, and the more they hinge forwards, the farther you will go forwards. Although not strictly a balance, this is a good neutral posture, linking naturally from twists to balances.

1 You have come up from the Revolved Triangle, so bend your knees in line with your toes, maintaining a lift in your tummy. Try not to stick your bottom out or to tuck it under. Use your thighs to hold you there and wait until they begin to burn.

2 Hinge forwards until your hands meet the floor and your chest is parallel to it. Your thighs should still be working. It is from these muscles that you slowly lift your bottom, lengthening the back of your legs. Keep your back long and your tummy pulled in.

3 Allow your upper body to relax. Feel the weight of the chest and head pull the lower spine long from the hips. The essence of a Forward Bend is to feel it within the backs of the legs. Let your head hang, while you push your seat bones up towards the ceiling.

incorrect The ability to touch the floor is worthy of praise, but not if it is achieved through back tension like this. Keep your back long by bending your knees and lifting your seat bones, or you will stretch the muscles of the back. (They are much smaller and tend to give way in the battle with the muscles in the backs of the legs.) Unlock your shoulders and use your thighs.

▶ **4** You can think of the head as a pendulum, hung from the hips via the spine, and here the picture gives a perfect example. Let the action of your heels pushing down and your buttocks going up leave your spine flowing down from your hips. Create as much space as you can between your legs and crotch for the hips to fold through as you bend over. Maintain the space in all your joints and enjoy letting your spine and hamstrings lengthen.

flying crow

Everyone falls over when they first try this posture, so you might as well resign yourself to the likelihood. If you are feeling brave but want some sort of soft landing, then practise in front of a cushion. Make sure you try it, for it is balance and not strength that is the key to the Flying Crow.

◀ **1** From the Triangle Forward Bend, bend the knees and start to raise the feet off the ground. If you feel that you have weak arms or are scared that you might fall flat on your face, then stay here. Lift up your heels and lift up your tummy. Your thighs will work hard but ignore them and concentrate on lifting your tummy so high that the legs begin to feel light. The more you lean forwards, the more you will find that the tummy pulls in.

▶ **2** A combination of leaning forwards to engage the stabilizing muscles of the back and a lot of tummy strength means that you can hang around in this posture for a while. The effort is felt in the tummy, but if the strength is not there you won't find yourself here. This is an example of balance through strength. It also shows you the lightness you should feel when performing the Flying Crow.

alternative 1 This picture shows a lower position in which more body weight is felt in the back of the arms. This will enable you to lift one foot tentatively off the floor. Make sure that you are looking forwards. This allows you to focus on the floor and reminds you of your balance. Pull your tummy in very tight as though it would lift straight through you. This will counter your impulse to collapse.

2 Once you find the balance point, the legs actually become quite light. This enables you to lift both legs up off the floor. Keep the shoulder blades open to make sure that both chest and back remain open. Lift your torso with your core strength at the same time – note the height of the tummy in this picture – rather than simply resting on your arms.

advanced If you keep lifting your tummy and the legs continue to be light, then you will find yourself in this position, the Handstand. Being upside down is so much fun and also very good for you. There are many reasons why inverting yourself may be good for you, but the best one is that it makes you feel like a child and reminds you of how much fun life can be. So even if you cannot suck yourself up to here by your tummy and back, then find a wall and play. If you do, remind yourself of how to keep your back open.

one-legged biceps curl

Balances are not easy, especially when you begin, because you feel as though something has been taken away from you. However, the mental and physical benefits you gain from their practice are far beyond the initial effort you may expend on learning them.

1 Having slowly rolled up to standing from Flying Crow, lift a leg and grab hold of the knee. Both hips and shoulders are even, although there is a great tendency to raise the hip and shoulder on the lifted side. Try and get the lovely long line in your collar bones.

▶ **2** One of the great things about yoga is the way it uses the body as its own personal gym machine. Here, you pull the knee high by using the biceps of the arms. As you do this, keep your shoulder blade wide and the elbow close to your side, as this will keep your shoulder blade flat to your ribs. This also has the effect of opening your chest. Notice that the head is right over the neck so that gravity goes straight through the body with the lowest possible resistance in the body.

incorrect Look how the leg is lifted by the top of the shoulder. This is intended to be a biceps curl, not a shrug and lift. Look how the hips are now uneven. If this happens to you, simply sit the raised sitting bone down and your hips will even out. Remember, balance is not just about remaining upright.

close-up This back view shows you how the action of curling your knee up can also teach you how to stabilize your shoulder blade. Keep your back broad and drop your shoulder blade so it feels as though that flat bone is curling under your armpit.

alternative If you really cannot balance in this posture, use a wall to steady yourself. Also, if you find that your hip is tight, then satisfy your need for knee height by stopping at parallel and concentrating on keeping your back long and upright. Pull your tummy in to help.

karate kid

This posture is a combination of strength and elegance, but at first it may feel ungainly and difficult. Try the easy version until you discover that your tummy and supporting hip take the strain, not the hip flexor of the lifted leg.

▶ 1 From One-legged Biceps Curl, lift your pubic bone up and lower your chest down to contract your tummy. Let go of the leg and pull your knee higher by pulling your tummy in harder. The effort should be in your tummy, not in your hip flexor. If you can find your balance here, drop your shoulder blades and lift your arms. You should feel the effort in the side of your waist and tummy. Let your supporting leg bend because that will help you to contact your middle. For the easy option stop at this point.

◀ 2 Look at the tummy – it is working hard to keep the leg up and straigtened. The more you pull your tummy in, lift your pubic bone and lengthen your leg, the longer and higher the extension will be. If you lower your arms as here, it will give you a chance to engage your back. This will help you to stabilize yourself and also give you a feeling of pushing up and off something as you find a lift.

close-up This close-up explains the emphasis on the tummy in this posture. Look at the groove on the side of the waist. That's where you will find the core or support muscles you need as opposed to using the hip flexors, which have the tendency to tighten your hips when you rely on them too much. It also means that you are more likely to extend your leg higher, which will make you feel even more graceful.

incorrect This method of Karate Kid is guaranteed to have your hip flexors flexing, since the entire weight of your leg is being held by them. Notice how the tummy is bulging. As a result of that bulge, the lower spine is once again called upon to hold up the body all by itself. Notice also how the lean backwards is preventing the tummy from being pulled in.

alternative As with the One-legged Biceps Curl, if you feel your balance is something to be worked on, use a wall to steady yourself. As you do so, use your other hand to feel how hard the hip flexor of the lifted leg is working (it will pop up like a cable). With your best endeavour, make your tummy pull in even harder. You may find that your leg will lift even higher as a result.

seated eagle

This posture is excellent for your insides, since they are flushed with blood in the action of squeezing your thighs together. After you have finished this posture, let yourself unwrap into the Tree, as you will now find it quite easy to balance and it helps to strengthen the hip further.

◀ **1** Bend the right knee, and cross the left leg over and tuck the toes behind. Cross the right arm over the left at the elbows, aiming the palms together. Push your elbows away from you and up to keep some space between your arms and your chest if you can. Keep the hips level and balanced.

▶ **2** To release the body, pull your tummy up and in, balancing on the straight leg. Unwrap your arms and drop your shoulder blades to lift them up. Place the previously crossing leg into a right angle to form a classic yoga shape, the Tree.

close-up It is not clear where the name Seated Eagle originated, but it does makes sense. You are "sitting" cross-legged, and the pretzel-like action of the arms opens your back and flares your shoulder blades – to spread your wings. The body should sit directly over your hips. Notice the light between the arms – try to keep the elbows up and the hands away from the body.

incorrect This is almost a "Seated Buzzard", with the curve in the middle and the hump in the back! If you collapse your middle and lean forwards, the head will still try to give you the impression that you are upright. Copy this and you will not feel the work of the posture in your thigh but feel as though you resemble a clumsy knot. Spread your wings and sit up. Don't slump.

alternative If you feel unsteady, then place your hands on your thighs and use your arms to help hold your spine long. Use the simplicity of this posture to keep your hips even and feel the work in your thigh.

rocket man

Practise this posture, taking time to repeat each leg, as through regular practice you will attain a good awareness of your hips, tummy and back. Also, through learning the feelings you gain in your body and replicating them into other postures, you will gain stability and understanding.

1 Balancing on one leg, use your arms to help stabilize your body on your bent supporting knee. Keep your shoulders down away from your ears and really extend backwards with your back leg. Think about lengthening your hip and thigh, as this will help you to feel the stretch from your stomach to your toes.

2 Notice that the chest is slightly above the hips. This allows the back to pull together, making it solid. The tummy is also pulled up to help stabilize the lower back. This also helps to steady the hip of the supporting leg. Really extend through your back leg as though you are pushing off to rocket forwards.

close-up You could call this posture "T", because ideally that is what it should look like. Keep your shoulders open away from your head and you should feel the muscles in the back engage to give you the lift you are looking for. Notice how the front ribs are closed to allow the spine to stretch its full length. The tummy is drawn in tight to support the lower spine and to help extend the back leg and open the hip. Try it, keeping your hips even.

incorrect More "Droopy" than Rocket, this is a common error. The mushroom back means the hips are the highest point, so the disengaged muscles lining the spine are working too hard. Push your back leg straight and lift your chest.

▶ **3** This is an enjoyable posture and this picture explains why. In Rocket Man you feel as though you are flying, with so much lightness in the hips that the supporting leg almost disappears. The body feels very long because of the simultaneous extension of the back leg backwards and the chest forwards. All the time the tummy is lifting up to let you feel a lightness, and the entire body begins to open. From here anything seems possible. Find your lightness and fly, even if you cheat by keeping one foot on the floor.

seated postures

When you get to the floor section you will need to remember not to collapse. Although a greater proportion of you rests on the floor, the increase in sensory response provided can give you even more of an idea of where your core is and how you lift. Always come to the floor exercises fresh. Feel your seat bones on the floor and lift your body up from them. Allow the hips to hinge; do not collapse them and bend from the spine. Most of all, remember that any Forward Bend comes from the hips, regardless of the length of the legs.

seated forward bend

You either love this posture or the back of your body complains so loudly that you don't. Be patient. Remember that the body must hinge in the middle, with both sides of the hinge as long as possible. To lie flat, the entire back of the body must be open.

▶ **1** Let your head relax so that your neck is long, and make your tummy as long as possible. After all, the longer the tummy, the longer your lower spine, and that means the deeper you hinge forwards. Think of lengthening your lower spine out of your hips, as opposed to dragging yourself forwards with your arms, and you'll find that any injury is very unlikely. You will also begin to understand more this feeling of a hinge. If you get the chance, ask someone to give you a push there. It's quite safe and feels lovely.

◀ **2** When you can, let the head bow and relax, as you did in the standing Forward Bend. Once again, you should feel that your spine is lengthening up, out and away from your hips. Extend your arms, relax and take time to breathe.

incorrect When people madly grab at their feet to show that they can touch their toes, it sometimes seems that if they let go, they would ping backwards owing to all the tension in their bowed spines. This posture is great as a back stretch, but as a Forward Bend not much of the body is going forwards and there is a big bend in the back. Since we spend so much time slouching over work, dinner or watching television, take this time to extend your spine and lengthen the backs of your legs.

alternative If you are not flexible, try this version and lift your chest as high up your thighs as possible. You will find a stretch in the back of your legs, even if your knees are as bent as you see here. Note how the length of the spine is mirrored by the length in the back of the thighs. Stay here, feeling the freedom of your spine and the stretch in your hips and hamstrings. Only when these lifting muscles are strong enough to counter the tightness in your legs will your hamstrings truly soften.

table

Have you ever seen a deck chair on a windy day, when its seat is blown through the frame? The Table should eventually have a similar feel, where the back muscles are "blowing" the front muscles open and up. Use your hands and feet to feel the floor and find the "lift".

◀ **1** The Table feels like a natural progression from a Seated Forward Bend, since all that opening needs consolidating. So sit up. Place your hands behind your bottom, slightly wider than shoulder width, which makes it easier to find your back strength until the flexibility of your shoulders appears. As you push up, keep your elbows soft and try to get your chest higher than your shoulders. Try to lengthen the front of your body, and you should find this helps to provide some more strength to stay up. If you find that dropping your head back all the way is difficult, either open your jaw wide or lengthen the back of your neck.

▶ **2** The Table is similar to the Side Triangle, in that you should feel as if you are making a tunnel underneath you. This means really having to find the muscles of your back, especially those that draw the shoulder blades down the back. When you find these, you will feel that they are responsible for lifting the chest higher and higher, opening the front of the shoulders and chest. So find the floor, push up and make a tunnel.

close-up The feet are the forgotten part of this posture – use them and they will help. If you have inflexible ankles, then really extend your toes to the floor, and not only will your ankles open but your arches will also improve. The more you can push down with your feet, the more you can engage the backs of the legs to help you lift. After all, they've been lengthened in the previous posture and now it is their chance to be strengthened in this one. Use your feet and feel the floor.

incorrect People execute this style of Table when they are unaware of their backs and of the fact that they have legs they can stretch. How many times when you've been slouched over your work do you push your chest up to release the tension you feel in it? Well this posture is exactly the same feeling. Get a neck, stop slouching, and you will understand how refreshed you can feel when you come down from the Table.

close-up Try not to lock your elbows, since this hyperextends them and takes the weight out of the muscles in the back and into your joints. If you can, keep working on getting your shoulder blades flat to your ribs, as this will really help to open your shoulders.

cobbler

This posture is also known as the Butterfly Hinge. Look at how the legs have opened right up, like wings. There is a lightness within the hips that allows this. Open the hips and revisit these postures as many times as necessary, to enable you to find this lightness in their separation.

1 Sit down from the Table and bring your heels towards your bottom as far as is comfortable. Holding your feet or ankles for support, lift your pubic bone up and try not to lean backwards. The higher you lift, the more your knees will spread apart.

2 From rolling back, pull your tummy up and in to lift you upright. As you do this, keep the feeling of separating the knees within your hips. These are separate and distinct sensations that do not seem to fit together, but practice will show that they do.

▶ **4** It may take a very long time for your hips to open sufficiently to allow your head to reach the floor, but wherever you get to in leaning forwards, remember that the more open your hips, the more space you have to roll forwards and through. Spend time getting your knees towards the floor before worrying yourself over how far you are from the floor. Spread your knees and hinge from the hips and your spine will look after itself.

3 If your inner thighs will not give in, use your arms to help maintain the length of your spine. Pulling the tummy up and in helps in two ways. It stops the lower spine collapsing and, second, the more you lift up, the more likely you will be able to release your inner thighs.

incorrect Look at the tension within the upper back during the struggle to get over the hips. As a result of this battle the inner thighs join in, resulting in the knees going up not down. This posture will only push tightness to where tightness already exists. Be alive and be intelligent. Feel the lift and begin to experience the opening of your body.

bridge

Think of the arc beneath a bridge – the smoother the arc, the stronger the structure. So when you attempt this posture, remember to keep as long an arc as possible in your back. This will prevent you from putting the bend on one part of the back, which always leads to discomfort.

1 From the Cobbler, lift your pubic bone up between your legs, and you'll find you begin to roll backwards. As your lower spine begins to near the floor, your legs will feel light enough to bring them into parallel lines with a nice bend in the knees. Keep lifting your pubic bone up to roll you down, and, as your spine unrolls on the floor, bring your heels as close to your bottom as is comfortable.

2 Once on the floor, lay your hands on either side of your body, pushing your forearms and hands down. This will help you to feel the muscles between your shoulder blades. Then press your heels down to feel the floor and keep rolling your pubic bone up between your legs. The thighs will feel the major work. If they don't, the lack of pubic lift will mean your lower back will begin to constrict.

close-up This angle is visually how you should feel. Just as in a standing Forward Bend, your hips are highest. Your thighs and hips are your strength. If you lift from them, you will find far less constriction in your back than if you struggle to lift with your arms. This entire sequence of photographs is one long roll of the pubic bone up between the legs.

3 If the posture in step 2 is very comfortable, then continue to lift your shoulder blades up off the floor and lift your pubic bone up between your legs. If in this higher posture you feel light, then take your right hand under your right shoulder and your left under your left. Stay here. Do not push with your arms. Keep lifting your middle, with the power in your thighs and the lift in your hips.

▶**4** The Bridge or the Big Back Bend has a status much the same as the Forward Bend or Handstand within a yoga class, for it shows everyone you have a flexible back. Try to think about being upside down, as if you have been walking on your hands and feet and a giant has turned you the wrong way up. This will make you feel as though you are pushing up not just with your arms but your legs and tummy as well. If you can play in this posture, move and sway. Try picking limbs up from the floor to reaffirm where your lift comes from. You are upside down, so be light-hearted and play.

double pigeon

The mechanics of this pose make it quite hard to strain and push, so in order to understand why this posture is so important, stay in it, rest in it and work intelligently within it. Be gentle with your body as, even though this posture feels lovely, going into it can elicit some strong feelings.

1 The action of placing one shin upon the other will, for some, be beyond the accommodation of their hips but if the shin does lie almost flat, then trust in your tummy strength and the hip will open up. As you sit there, sit as tall out of your hips as is possible.

2 Push your top knee down (in the Assembly position, both knees) and lift your pubic bone between your legs. You will feel the tummy pull in and the knees spread. Do not lean backwards, just roll your hips up and back. Stay here and feel the spread in the legs.

advanced If your hips do not feel the desired deep stretch with your shins lying on each other, then pull your knees so that they are inside your ankles and you will find the depth of sensation you have been looking for. Breathe slowly and deeply, emphasizing the exhale to help you let go of the tension in those deep muscles.

alternative If when you try and place your shin on top of the other, your body prevents your leg from moving or the knee sticks up high in the air, or your ankle and foot feel as though they are going to snap, then move into the Assembly position sitting with simple crossed-legs.

▶ **3** Keep sucking your tummy in and up until you feel your hips begin to roll forwards. Keep rolling them forwards, up and over your legs, until you find yourself over your legs. Push your bottom down and back, pull your tummy in and up and lift your chest up by using the muscles of your upper back. This will extend your spine and allow you to find space within your hips and lower spine.

batfink

In this posture you wrap your arms around your legs as though you were cloaking them in bat wings. This will keep your back open and broad while you curl your pubic bone up and draw your knees to your chest by pulling your tummy away from your thighs.

▶ 1 Start by balancing on your bottom and, while maintaining your balance, learn to curl your pubic bone up and your tail between your legs, as this is the beginning of extending your spine into a long, smooth "C" shape. You have to hold this "C" shape in order to have a smooth roll from bottom to shoulders and back up again. Let your arms go forwards and your chest backwards since this will help you round and open your upper spine. You do not want to throw yourself up and down with the momentum from your legs, so spend some time here until you feel that you have the smoothest "C" back you can possibly get.

◀ 2 Rolling back and up is fun. You get a lovely feeling of massaging the muscles along your back and the impression that you are a child's toy. The art of rolling back and up lies in your pubic lift, as this will keep any gaps or holes in your spine from appearing, in other words, any part of your back that does not wish to roll with the rest of your back on the floor. Notice how the body is still in exactly the same position even though it has been turned on to the space between the shoulder blades.

advanced If you have rolled back and forth quite happily and fancy a challenge, try recreating a Forward Bend while balancing on your bottom. Enter Batfink as in step 1, then slowly pull your bent knees as close to your shoulders as you can. Lift the arms and straighten your legs by using the muscles in the front of your thighs. Try it out. Play one leg at a time.

alternative If there is no way your spine will allow you to roll back and forth, assume this position. Keep lifting your pubic bone into your tummy, while keeping the knees relaxed above your hips. This will strengthen your abdomen and allow you eventually to roll through the hips.

incorrect Look here at how the chest is lifted and the tummy is forced to bulge out, leaving more weight to be carried in the lower back. Also, the hip flexors are the main muscle holding the knees high. When these tighten they pull the hip girdle forwards with them and, since your hips are attached to your spine, this means a more pronounced hollow in your lower back. Don't allow feeling tall in the posture to come at the expense of being tight. Besides, straight lines don't roll.

tortoise

Achieving this posture takes patience and time. When inside it at your limit, slow down and take time. Come out as if coming out of hibernation, for if you move quickly, you will miss great subtleties and sensations. The Tortoise can unlock the deep places where we store our tension.

▶ **1** The Tortoise posture is all about coming forwards. Just as a tortoise extends its head out of its protective shell, you have to figure out how to pull your body up and forwards out of your hips. Put your arms under your bent legs and extend forwards. The posture demonstrated here is more than deep enough for most people, since it requires you not only to roll your hips forwards between your legs but also to extend your spine forwards and up from your rolled hips. The result is an intense sensation in the hips and lower spine.

◀ **2** This is a real challenge since both your legs and your body have to go forwards away from your hips. The arms extend backwards, away from the head. This is going beyond the Forward Bend you are used to, since you have to take your body beneath your legs. However, remember that the bend originates inside the hips, not through dragging your spine between your legs. Whatever you do, keep your back long and take time to feel the groin open up to give the hips space to move through.

incorrect A classic posture of the head bound student, this method of performing the Tortoise will inevitably end with you on your back. The body is collapsing forwards, beginning with the shoulders and moving all the way down the back. Although the hips may feel the stretch, they will not stretch far because of the distinct lack of support from the rest of the body. Be patient and you will win in the end.

alternative If your hips allow for very little play, follow this example. Use your arms as struts to help lengthen and lift your spine up and out of your hips. Not only will this feel more comfortable, but it will also put you in touch with the tummy lift. This lift, when strong enough, will allow your muscles around the hip joint to soften so that the hips can then hinge closer to the thighs. If you find yourself here, then you need to pay more attention to all the Forward Bend exercises.

advanced If your hips and spine allow, proceed forwards and down, rolling your palms up to the ceiling (thumbs facing in) so you can try to grab hold of your bottom or clasp hands. The idea is that through slotting your shoulder blades under your knees, the knees can act as a weight to push your body lower. Clasping the hands on the lower spine then provides some sensations you can respond to and lift away from. Extend your body as long as you can along the floor and you will feel all the tension release from your tail.

shoulder stand

There are many benefits to practising inverted postures, primarily because it flushes the head and neck with a large supply of blood. This not only helps to relax you and release tension from your head and neck, but may also leave you feeling clearer and fresher than when you began.

1 Lift your pubic bone up into your tummy until your legs are rolling over your head. Lift your shoulder blades up off the floor. Any neck pain should disappear when you work the back muscles hard to lift the shoulder blades up off the floor.

2 If resting your knees on your head strains your back, try this version, as it demands a long spine. Basic rules: if your neck hurts, then lift your shoulder blades up off the floor. If your spine or lower back hurts, then take your hips backwards away from your head.

alternative Roll backwards into an "L". Bend the knees as you need to. Pull the abdomen in, brace the floor with your arms and draw your shoulder blades down your body away from your ears. Menstruating women will benefit from staying in this posture. If you really want to relax then put your legs up against a wall.

advanced Attempt this posture only if you are fully aware of your tummy and back core muscles. If you are, then you will find it. If not, don't try it. It is fun and the key is found between your shoulder blades.

▶**3** Follow the same two rules. If your neck hurts and feels tight, lift your shoulder blades up and away from the floor. (Persistent pain means don't be silly, stop doing it and seek advice.) Second, if your lower spine aches, then take your hips back away from your head. Then warm your kidneys with your hands and stay there, constantly feeling the lift, for as long as you feel comfortable. There are many benefits, so practise and learn to feel them. Please note that women are not advised to practise inverted postures during the first three days of menstruation.

fish to corpse

These three postures flow into each other and lead you into a deeper state of relaxation. The Fish helps you extend and open the front of your body. The Baby pose helps you be aware of the expansion of your spine and the freedom of your hips. Corpse lets you become aware of this space.

◀ **1 fish** This a classic counter pose to end with after a Shoulder Stand. The reason why can be seen in the neck. Having compressed the front of the neck and lengthened the back, the pushing of the elbows down and the arching of the upper back can allow you to drop your head right back until the top of your head rests on the floor. Remember to stretch your legs and lengthen your tummy, so that you feel as though the arch in the top of your body is grounded in the rest of it. As you do this, try not to make the arch come solely from your lower spine, as this may make your back ache when you slowly lower yourself down. Most of all, open your chest. Breathe into the space between your shoulder blades and, as you breathe out, lengthen your waist.

▶ **close-up** This angle shows the positioning of the hands and that the emphasis is most certainly found in lifting and opening the chest. See if you can find out how to arch your upper back without having to overarch your lower back. Breathe deeply into the top of your chest and open the space between your shoulders.

2 baby If you find your lower back aches at any point at the end, come into the Baby pose. Use this posture to find out just how long your spine can get. Ground your sacrum and coccyx on the floor while pulling your knees down into your armpits, as this will open your hips and flatten your lower spine. Make sure that your ribs do not stick up, as this will leave you with a hollow under your ribs, and keep your shoulders away from your head.

3 From the Baby you know it is time to relax, so lower both heels to the floor with a bend in the knees. This should make sure that your spine feels long and flat on the floor.

4 Let one leg go straight, but as you do so, notice how much of your spine pulls up and off the floor. This is owing to tension in the front of your hip. Allow your leg to let go and the spine to remain soft.

5 corpse When you feel ready, allow your other leg to go straight and, once again, watch how the spine lifts. If your lower spine hurts with both legs down, then return to both legs bent and heels on the floor. Let go and be prepared to spend some time here.

chilling out

There is no question that when you're tired you want to rest and that after resting you'll feel better. Another simple fact is that when your muscles are relaxed, you tend to feel relaxed in your head too. When you have finished your practice, you may well find that you feel tired.

◀ **1** Try lying on your front with the soft parts of your body on the floor. You'll discover that it is very easy to find this sinking feeling when there are no bony parts of you causing discomfort. We come back to the scientific law that states that for each action, there is an equal and opposite reaction. So, the harder you work, the better you'll rest. When you know just where the tired muscles are, it is easier to relax them. Equally, the harder they work, the easier it is to get them to relax. What you end up with is a body ready and willing to relax. If you repeat this regularly, you will learn to know the feeling of letting go. Eventually this awareness will be with you all the time, not just after exercise.

▶ **2** Roll on to your back and keep that feeling of sinking that you found on your tummy and let your body go "splat", including your bony parts. Check your hips are open and your shoulder blades are broad and allow your chest to open. Let go, it's the end.

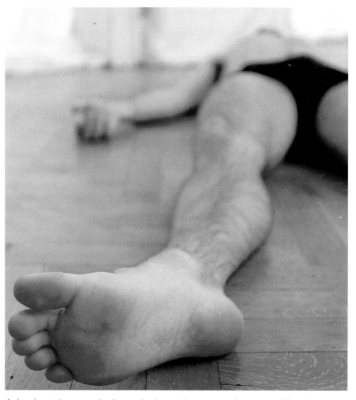

3 As you lie there, you will want to think and be active in your head. So get as far away from your head as you can by finding and mentally feeling your feet with your consciousness. Physically do nothing and mentally take a holiday to your toes. Your mind will want you to fidget, move, think or imagine. It will cling madly on to any source of entertainment, even down to counting your breathing or heart rate.

4 Against the wandering mind, you have an advantage. You have your body beneath you, with its many thousands of impulses and sensations. If your mind wants to be busy, entertain it by watching, living, the sensations of you. This is true relaxation, meditation, chilling out – whatever you want to call it. But most of all, the beauty is that everything you've been wanting – release, a source of wellbeing – is you. Let go and feel.

sequences

There are three warm-up sequences here, and four routines. You do
not need to copy everything you see, but practise what you can.
If you like, refer back to the main page for each posture for more
details. Spend time in each of the postures to see how your breathing
affects them, or flow between them with only one breath held in each.
Try spending at least ten breaths in each posture in one practice and
then only one in another, as this will build endurance and
cardiovascular fitness respectively. At the end of each sequence, make
time for five minutes of stillness.

PUTTING IT TOGETHER

Look at a river and you will see that in the middle its current runs fast, taking all the sediment it carries far down towards the sea. Look now at the sides or the banks of the river and you will see the current moving slower, eddying and playing with the sediment it carries and laying it down on the banks. This build-up of deposits will eventually lead to a change in the shape of the river as it begins to push the fast-flowing centre farther and farther away from it.

FAT, THE RIVER AND YOU

Your body is one big river of energy. Wherever there is poor circulation, sediment (or fat) will build up, and when it does, not only the inside but also the outside will show this. If you sit down, remaining static and inactive, it is common sense that you will not feel or look in prime physical condition. After all, your muscles, which act as pumps, are not active to help your river keep flowing freely inside you, and build-up will occur.

To help you find your river and help activate

these natural pumps, put together all that you've learnt so far: hinging through your hips from ape to man to find the "pumps" in your buttocks and thighs, using your back and tummy to keep your spine long and free.

Think of all you learn and read in here as a map. But make sure that at every stage you ask yourself "Does this map make sense to me?" If it doesn't, don't hesitate to discard it and start again. If it does make sense, then follow and feel so you find these words, actions, postures and descriptions making sense in your body. Listen and feel until they become a physical sensation.

WARMING UP

On the following pages are some simple warm-up sequences. All of them are flowing, which means no postures are held for long; they simply flow as the breath does, from inhale to exhale, standing to bending, looking up to stepping back. All the time you are doing them, make sure that your spine is long, your tummy is engaged and your neck is soft from the shoulder blades going down and out, not up and in.

If you can't do this, return to the beginning and relearn where your core strength is. Remember, too, that you don't move just during the 10 or 15 minutes of this routine, so why apply these rules only for the duration of your practice? When you drive a car, are your shoulder blades up around your ears because of stress? If so, get them down. When you are standing at the sink or cooking, is your spine long and your tummy pulled in to support your lower spine? When you sit at your office desk, can you find the lift up and off the chair? If you become more aware, you will find that all movement will begin to feel easier.

left and right The exercises here can teach you to find your core strength and the lunges and standing postures will help increase your stamina. However, you need to put this information to good use in the rest of your life as well, not just when you are being "fit", and then you will really feel it.

relaxing sequence – warm-up 1

This is a relaxing warm-up to try before moving on to the later postures. This way, the muscles will be primed and know what to expect, lessening the chance of injury. These movements are intended to flow, one into the other, so don't hold each one for long, maybe 30 seconds or two

1 lying down Begin by lying on your back with your arms at your sides. Use your senses to discover how much of you rests flat on the floor, and every time you exhale see if you can release down a little more.

2 upper back arch As you breathe in, direct your breath to the top part of your chest and see if through contracting your upper back – the muscles that line the spine in between your shoulder blades – you are able to lift up your breastbone.

3 softened chest As you breathe out, soften your chest so that the upper back arch is allowed to soften. Repeat these actions so that your upper back begins to be more mobile. See if you can feel just your upper back moving.

7 both knees to chest Slowly pull both knees to your chest. Drag your heels to your bottom before you lift your legs, as this will allow you to maintain a stable core, as opposed to your back having to arch or your abdomen bulge.

8 letter "L" The straightness of your legs is secondary to the feeling of work in your core and stability in your hips. It doesn't matter whether your legs are straight; keep your back long along the floor. Feel as though you are stretching the back of your body. Breathe and lengthen your body.

9 lowering the legs Begin lowering both legs by bending and separating your knees, while simultaneously lifting your pubic bone. This will mean that you are using primarily your core strength to lower your legs.

deep breaths. The whole sequence will take only a few minutes, but the benefits of doing it regularly will soon show in the way that your core strength is improved, and all kinds of movements, not just the ones in this book, will become easier.

4 knee up to chest After resting for a few moments, exhale deeply. Lift one leg up into your chest, clasping your hands just below your knee. Keep both sides of your waist long and see if you can lengthen your buttocks and lower spine.

5 submarine Let go of the knee and extend your leg. If your leg cannot straighten, then keep your knee bent and push your heel high. The key here is not to let your tummy bulge up and your lower back arch off the floor. Keep pulling your ribs and stomach away from the upright leg.

6 lowering the leg Lower the leg with a bend in the knee and the leg slightly turned out, or straight. Maintain the strength in your tummy so that neither your back arches nor your tummy bulges up. Repeat with the other leg.

10 roll up Once your feet have reached the floor, allow your legs to roll away from each other fully and pull your tummy up and in so hard that you end up looking through your legs. Follow this pull and roll up to sitting.

11 roll over Be aware of the movement of your hips as you roll up. As you roll over your legs, do so with your hips and not simply by leaning forwards from your lower spine. Learn to hinge forwards, so repeat rolling back and forth until you can really feel the movement of your hips.

12 corpse Finally, roll back, doing so along your entire spine. When on the floor, slowly extend one leg, then the other, and rest. Use your senses to see if any more of your body is resting on the floor than when you began.

resting rocket man – warm-up 2

This sequence is all based upon activity and release, so when being active, really use your muscles to make you feel as though you are flying through the poses. Then, when you enter the Child poses they will feel like home since your muscles will be crying out for some rest and this will help

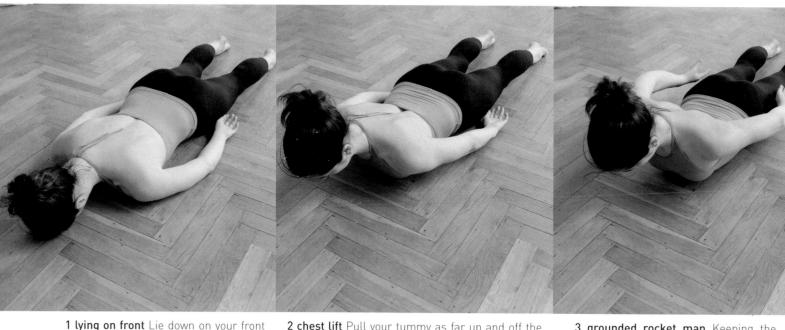

1 lying on front Lie down on your front and concentrate on the soft parts of your body on the floor (tummy, thighs and chest). Try to relax until you feel as though as much as possible of the front of you is touching the floor.

2 chest lift Pull your tummy as far up and off the floor as possible to keep your lower spine in place and lengthen the front of your body from your chest to your forehead. Keep your shoulder blades open and arms relaxed, as they were in the previous posture.

3 grounded rocket man Keeping the back of your neck long, your tummy up and your legs relaxed, lift your elbows up until your thumbs meet the creases under your buttocks. Make sure you leave your shoulder blades open.

7 double leg lift To lift both legs is tricky without drooping your lower spine or collapsing your chest, so pay attention to those details as opposed to the height of your legs off the floor.

8 big-belly child Again, use your abdomen to stop your back collapsing as you push yourself back. The wider your knees, the more open your hips will feel, but if your lower back feels tight, try belly gazing which will help to free any tension.

9 elbows Resting your head on your thumbs, keep your navel the highest point underneath you. Make a long, smooth arc from head to toe to let the strength of your front open your back.

you let your muscles relax further into the pose. Since it does not take long, try repeating it until your body seems to flow through the sequence with your muscles smoothly taking you from one pose to the next. Repeated regularly, you will really start to feel the benefits in your core strength.

4 child Place your hands under your shoulders and pull your tummy firmly up and in. This will brace your back as you push your bottom towards your heels. If your shoulders are very tight, take your arms into a wide "Y".

5 belly gazing Return to the starting position before finding this pose and see if you are any more relaxed than before. Then, placing your hands beneath your forehead, push your elbows down and gaze down at your abdomen, feeling it pull up and in.

6 leg lift Keep your posture the same: open back, long and lifted front, long lower spine. Lift one leg by lengthening your thigh back and away from you. Remember to try squeezing the top of that leg's buttock. Change legs.

10 naughty child This encourages you to push your bottom in the air. Think of a long arch from your bottom to your fingertips – let the length in the back reflect the length of your front.

11 press up Ideally your shoulders are directly over your wrists, with a big space beneath you. Push your chest up off the floor to open the space between your shoulder blades and once again find the arc from your forehead to your toes.

12 lying on front See how far you can let go into the floor; how much more of your front touches the floor than when you began. Consciously contract a group of muscles, then release and relax them.

standing sequence – warm-up 3

This warm-up allows you to take all that you have learnt about your body so far and apply it to a standing stance. We spend most of our waking life in an upright posture, so it makes sense that we practise something that mimics the patterns of our everyday life or we stand little chance of

1 standing Stand tall with your chest lifted, hands by the sides, and as you stand, feel the connection from the heels to the back of your head. Draw the shoulder blades out and down. Soften the chest as you exhale.

2 lifting arms Inhale. Feel the connection between your arms and your back and lift the arms as you drop the shoulder blades, so the shoulders are relaxed and down. Take the arms forward, so you can feel the movement of the shoulder blades, then bring both arms above your head.

3 forward bend Exhale. Soften your knees and lift the bottom so you can lengthen the abdomen and spine. This will ensure that you hinge forwards from the hips, rather than collapse through the lower spine.

7 single leg stretch Exhale. Use your hips as a hinge to simultaneously push the front leg long and lower the torso over the front leg. Enjoy the stretch but keep some softness in your front knee. Do not hyperextend your knee.

8 looking up forward bend Inhale. Step forwards, placing your feet together. Try to do this by bending your back leg. As you step you will really feel the hip of the straight leg. See if you can keep some lightness in your body as you make this move. You may have to make two smaller steps.

9 forward bend Exhale. Push your heels down, keeping the knees soft, lift the bottom, pull the tummy up and in and let the head relax and drop down to the feet. Place your palms flat on the floor either side of your feet.

changing our habitual patterns of movement. Perform this warm-up until it makes sense, and you can really let your breath take you from one posture to the next. When you have achieved this, try to discover a feeling of light-footedness, so that when you move you are in full control.

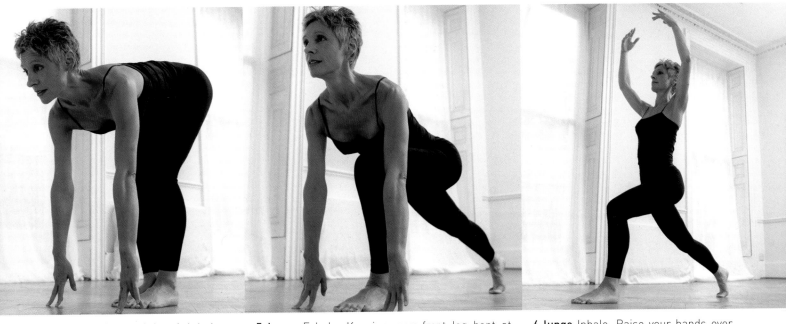

4 looking up forward bend Inhale. Using your upper back rather than the neck, look up and open the ribs so that you will have more room to inhale. Lengthen the stomach and keep lifting your bottom to the ceiling.

5 lunge Exhale. Keeping your front leg bent at 90 degrees, lunge the other leg backwards, really concentrating on lengthening your leg right up through the abdomen. Keep the hips above the level of the knees, meanwhile keeping the muscles of the stomach strong.

6 lunge Inhale. Raise your hands over the head. Lift up through the hips and keep the lower spine long by lifting your pubic bone. Keep the back leg long and straight, and feel the sensations happening in your hips.

10 flat back to lifting arms Inhale. Look up and extend your spine. Soften the knees and pull the tummy in, so you can hinge up to standing through your hips while maintaining a long spine. Drop the shoulders to lift the arms.

11 standing Exhale. Relax your chest as you breath out, so you feel the weight of your arms between the shoulder blades. Remember to take your arms in front of the body to keep the shoulder blades flat to the ribs. Repeat on the other side to make one round of this sequence.

earthing sequence

When you are tired, stressed or anxious, getting close to the floor and truly feeling it can allow your breath and emotions to calm down. Use this sequence to learn where the floor is and how you tense muscles unnecessarily while performing the simplest of postures.

1 sleeping superman Lie on the floor and try to feel yourself free-falling through the floor. Play with the upper back and shoulder blades. This will help you to feel the back open up.

2 child Breathe and take your time. Use the tummy and back to help you move between this and the posture in the previous picture.

3 cobbler Push yourself all the way back on to your bottom. Keep the hips low and feel the buttocks stretch. Use these muscles to help to separate your knees.

7 knee hug Lower your hips slowly so that you know where the weight of the body is. Keep your awareness in the hips as you hug the knees. Lengthen the lower spine.

8 single leg "L" Lay one leg flat, really stretching through the hip as you lengthen the other leg towards the ceiling. Keep the weight inside the hips. Relax the chest and keep the tummy in.

9 single knee hug As you bend the knee in the air, feel the buttocks and your lower spine lengthen. Do not lose this sensation, but really savour it. Repeat on the other side from single leg "L".

4 letter "L" Squeeze your buttocks to open the legs, then lift the pubic bone to help you roll along the spine to form the shape of the letter "L". If you are inflexible, you may find it necessary to bend your knees.

5 batfink Hold on to the back of the knees to help you begin rolling and make sure you roll through all of the spine, without holes or bumps.

6 bridge Roll up to Cobbler and then, with your feet ready, roll the spine down and lift the hips up in the air. Keep the work in the hips so the spine stays long.

10 upper back bow Lower both legs to the floor, keeping the weight of them inside the hips and abdomen so that the lower back stays long. Separate the shoulders and lengthen the upper spine along the floor.

11 upper back arch Soften your chest and contract the shoulders down and out to feel the neck lengthen and the middle and upper back arch.

12 corpse Release and relax the muscles you have just worked. Feel them soften into the floor and, once again, try to free-fall through the floor. Let the earth hold you up.

energizing sequence

To energize, you have to get everything moving, so this sequence is composed of big postures requiring large movements to flow between them. Within the space of these movements you can really begin to feel the body beneath you. Take your time getting from one posture to the next.

1 lunge After performing up to five single leg lunges, stay in the Lunge and really push the back leg straight. Keep the work in the hips by lifting the tummy.

2 pert buttocked warrior Roll the hip of the back leg around, while keeping the front knee still. Let the arms drop to shoulder height, but keep their weight in between the shoulder blades.

3 triangle Push the front leg straight and use that hip as a hinge to rotate the torso towards the ground. Use the tummy to keep the chest and hips rolled at an angle of 90 degrees to the floor.

7 forward bend When you have completed the postures on both sides, jump forwards and, with soft knees, push the heels down while at the same time lifting the bottom.

8 karate kid Roll up to standing and bring your beginning lunge leg with you. Contract the tummy backwards, so that you feel the weight of the leg in the stomach muscles.

9 rocket man Take that leg backwards in line with your body and really stretch that leg through the sensations you felt in Rocket Man.

4 dog split Use the tummy and back hip to roll the chest parallel to the floor. Pushing your hands flat, kick the back leg straight behind you so it makes a line with the wrist.

5 up dog Slowly lower yourself into the Press Up position and, with both feet on the floor, drop the hips and lift the chest. Use the back, keep it open and draw the shoulders down.

6 down dog Lift back into Press Up position from your tummy. Continue to lift the tummy as you separate the shoulders while pushing the bottom back and up. Lunge the other leg forwards and repeat.

10 thigh lunge Bend the supporting knee and stretch your back, lowering yourself into this knee trembling pose. Make sure you keep the abdomen high, off the front thigh.

11 revolved triangle Take the opposite hand alongside the front foot and lift the bottom up with the other hand. This will twist you towards the leg, but use the tummy to help twist you around. Via Press Up, Up Dog, Down Dog and a Jump, go back to Rocket Man on the other leg.

12 triangle forward bend Finish with another Press Up, Up Dog and Down Dog sequence, and then jump straight into this posture. Keep the knees soft and lift the bottom. Finish with some relaxing postures and stillness.

strength sequence

Although this sequence seems to rely on arm strength, the strength you need is in fact to be found in your core. When you begin the first posture, try to feel the weight of your body being carried within your back and stomach, rather than in your shoulders and arms.

1 press up Keep the navel high underneath you and draw the shoulder blades down the back. Then bend the elbows (do not collapse) and, as you exhale, relax the chest so that your full weight is felt in the back.

2 up dog Drop your hips and lift the chest with the muscles you used in the Press Up. Stretch the legs through the tummy back to the toes.

3 down dog Using your tummy and stopping briefly in top Press Up, lift the hips into Down Dog. Pay careful attention to the feelings in the wrists, shoulders and tummy.

7 side triangle Roll on to the outside of the back foot and roll on to your side, so the top leg remains in the air. See if you can grab hold of that top big toe without crushing the space underneath you.

8 jump Jump into Lunge on the other side and repeat from the Lunge to the Dog Split and Side Triangle on the other side. Then, after completing both sides, jump both feet to behind the wrists, drop your head and lift your bottom. Release any tension from your lower spine.

9 triangle forward bend Feel the tummy pull up and in as you lift your bottom. Pay attention to this lift.

4 jump Having felt the strength through your wrists, shoulders and tummy, keep it strong as you jump up. At the top of the jump, take one foot forward, ready for the Lunge.

5 lunge Keep light in this posture, as if you are still in the top of the Jump. Use the back to hold the arms up and the tummy to hold you buoyant from the hips.

6 dog split In one smooth move, push the front leg all the way back in a Dog Split, but keep the shoulders and hips even to maintain the strength of the posture in your core.

10 flying crow Place your knees on the back of the arms, lift the heels and find that lift. It feels as though a rope around your waist is holding you up.

11 handstand (advanced flying crow) Press your hands down, contract the back and let the lift straighten you out. Practise this posture separately, against a wall if you wish, but continue to feel the lift from your middle.

12 press up Using the shoulder girdle as a hinge, and keeping the arms strong, let yourself drop back into a Press Up. Omit this posture if you are not sure of your ability. Relaxation and stillness must follow this sequence.

relaxing sequence

The postures are all designed to get your hips level – or above your head. Inversion takes a great strain from your heart and provides your head with an amount of blood that gravity denies you. With the release of tension from your shoulders and neck, this will leave you feeling lighter.

1 seated forward bend Remember that a forward bend does not automatically require straight legs. Hinge from the hips and lengthen the tummy up and out of the hips.

2 table Take your hands back behind you and, keeping the back open, use your bottom and back to lift you into the Table. Soften the chest to feel the stretch in the chest and the shoulders.

3 cobbler Lower your bottom down and draw the heels towards the crotch. Use your bottom to open the knees towards the floor and hinge forwards through the hips.

7 tortoise Roll up and separate the legs, so that you can hinge through them. Remember, the object is to open the hips and lower spine, not to straighten the legs.

8 shoulder stand Roll down and make the letter "L" with your legs in the air. Pull your knees and shins towards your face to help you engage the abdomen.

9 batfink Roll down to an "L" again and pause momentarily before rolling any residual tension from the back and spine. Take your time and roll as slowly as you can.

4 bridge Roll the spine back on to the floor and continue rolling the hips up into this back bend. Keep the hips long and learn how you can lengthen the lower spine in this pose.

5 double pigeon Come down slowly, choose a leg to cross on top or in front and hinge forwards to open up the hip and lower spine. Change legs.

6 batfink Draw both knees towards the shoulders, while curling the lower spine so you engage the tummy and roll fluently down and up along the spine.

10 fish Having felt your spine open and bow, lie down to remind yourself of the muscles of the upper back. Arch the upper spine by drawing the shoulder blades wide and then down the back.

11 baby Bend your knees to bring the legs up to the chest. Bend the knees so you can push your bottom away from you along the floor. Once again, you feel the hips and lower spine open.

12 corpse Take the heels down to the floor and rest with the knees still up before relaxing fully with the legs down. Give the back plenty of time to adjust to its new length.

INDEX

acknowledgements and addresses

AUTHOR'S ACKNOWLEDGEMENTS
Thank you to the space above my mat. Mum and
Dad. Julia. Carly. Lesley. Friends, for without you
the world seems hard work. Students and all
those who continue to show me all that I'm too
close to see. The publisher, and my editor Katy,
for this opportunity. Play well.
JONATHAN MONKS

PUBLISHER'S ACKNOWLEDGMENTS
Many thanks to Judith Kleinman for allowing us
to use the space at Highbury to shoot the
photographs.

USEFUL ADDRESSES
Danceworks
16 Balderton Street
London W1K 6TN
(Opposite Selfridges Clock)
tel: 020 7629 6183
email: info@danceworks.co.uk
www.danceworks.co.uk

The British Wheel of Yoga
25 Jermyn Street
Sleaford
Lincs. NG34 7RU
tel: 01529 306 851
email: office@bwy.org.uk
www.bwy.org.uk

Yoga Therapy Centre
90-92 Pentonville Road
London N1 9HS
tel: 020 7689 3040
email: enquiries.yogatherapy@virgin.net
www.yogatherapy.org

Health and Fitness Solutions Ltd
The City of London Medical Centre
Lower Ground Floor, 11-13 Crosswalls
London EC3N 2JY
tel: 020 7702 1112
www.hfs.uk.net

for listings of yoga institutes in Canada and US:
www.yogadirectory.com; www.jivamuktiyoga.com